WHAT PEOPLE ARE SAYING

"A beautifully written book told straight from the heart with honest vulnerability."
-Tiffani Freckleton RN, NTMC.
Best-selling author

"This book is powerful, informative and filled with heartfelt personal experiences. ... Brita's faith, prayer, and forgiveness become her source of strength, and she regains her health and happiness of life."
-Toni Stone Bruce
Author/Motivational Speaker
Precious Stones 4 Life, LLC

"I found a hard-won tale about learning how to recognize the beauty throughout the brutal journey-not just at the end."
- Danny Kutz

"Brita has a talent for sharing the raw parts of her health journey in such an authentic way that it allows her readers to be more accepting of themselves."
-Pualei Lynn
Owner of EDYNKEI Boutique & Founder of ELEVATE Women's Group

"I was drawn into this book and Brita's story from the first page.... I was riveted to her story and read through this book in one sitting. I highly recommend it!"
-Becky Peyton
doTERRA wellness advocate

"This book was a great read!. This book is raw and real!. I recommend this book to anyone that is in need of a new perspective on hardships, struggles, and life in general!"
- Heather Peterson

"Everyone needs to read this book! I could not put this book down and felt every triumph and pain with her as the story progressed."
-Aubin Palmer
Business and Life Coach
Aubin Palmer Coaching

"What if you lived a lifestyle of beating, ignoring, and reducing your body into a state of chronic illness? In Getting Through Today, Brita Peterson tells her story of living with chronic sickness and moving from surviving to thriving by trusting her intuition and faith."
-Maureen Ryan Blake
Maureen Ryan Blake Media Production

"Her words provide a strong and understanding perspective for anyone who's facing their own health obstacles or re-conceptualizing their dreams."
-Shelby Kottemann
2x Internationally Bestselling Author, Intuitive Healer, Artist

GETTING

How Chronic Illness Taught Me

THROUGH

The Beauty in Being Broken

TODAY

BRITA BIGLER PETERSON

GETTING THROUGH TODAY
How Chronic Illness Taught Me the Beauty in Being Broken

Copyright © 2023 by Brita Peterson

Inspired Legacy Publishing is a division of (DBA) Inspired Legacy, LLC
PO Box 900816
Sandy UT 84090-0816.

Changing Names & Medical Advice
Some names and identifying details have been changed to protect the privacy of individuals.
This book is not intended as a substitute for the medical advice of physicians. The reader
should regularly consult a physician in matters relating to his/her health and particularly
with respect to any symptoms that may require diagnosis or medical attention.

ISBN 979-8-9871952-0-8 (paperback)
ISBN 979-8-9871952-1-5 (hardcover)

Printed in the United States of America.

CONTENTS

ACKNOWLEDGMENTS

I am eternally grateful for my husband, Jeff, for loving me through all of the ups and downs. I could not have gotten through all of these struggles without his kindness and patience. I feel so blessed to have such an amazing man by my side.

My beautiful children, Landan, Taylor, Callen, Carter and Avery, are my favorite people in the whole world and I am so grateful for their love, compassion and strength. I am in awe of the people they are and I am so proud to be their mom.

Thank you to all of my wonderful family and friends who have supported me through this journey. I could not have survived without each and every one of you.

Of course, this book wouldn't be what it is without Bridget Cook Burch, who helped me find my voice and taught me how to write my authentic story; Hannah Lyon, who stuck with me through many rewrites and always had the best suggestions and encouragement; and Rebecca Hall Gruyter, for taking a chance on me and believing in my story.

Thank you to Alli Reid for the cover photo. It was such a fun photoshoot!

INTRODUCTION

Sharing my story hasn't been an easy or short journey. In fact, it's been really hard and has taken so much time and I've wondered many times along the way if I should even do this.

You might wonder in the first few chapters what my story has to do with being broken, because I had a happy childhood where I grew into a competitive athlete who was motivated and strong. I share these first parts with you so you can see where I started and see the dynamic person I was. In order to see how broken I began to feel, you will need to see the gradual decline of my sparkly and vibrant demeanor—to see how far down I began to sink into my mind and my body and was no longer the happy, strong person I used to be.

Chronic health and mental illness plagued my body and I battled with myself for years, trying to get back to the person I was. But I found that I would never be back to the person I used to be, instead, I learned a depth and a power in myself that I never would have found had I not gone through so many trials. Even though I have not seen all of the beauty along the way during these dark times, I can see it now. And I have been able to redefine myself into a stronger, more compassionate version of myself that I like even better than the old version.

I have found strength in myself to keep fighting and now I want to give hope to others going through similar things. I would like to reach those dark places you may be sitting in and give you hope for your future, knowing that you can continue to get through today.

Below are the lyrics to a song I have written that tells my story and I hope you can come along and be broken with me, showing up as you are, the beautiful, messy, amazing person you are right now.

BEAUTIFUL BROKEN
© 2022 BRITA PETERSON

I'm tired of pretending, so tired of acting strong.
I found myself in pieces, they tell me broken is wrong.

A girl with all the big dreams, I'm no longer playing small.
Everything I'm hiding is exposed through shattered walls.

Beautiful broken, gather up the pieces.
Much stronger rewritten. Beautiful broken.

I feel destroyed and fallen while knowing things should change.
I mend my aching heart while fighting through the pain.

Beautiful broken, gather up the pieces.
Much stronger rewritten. Beautiful broken.

Come together. Be broken with me. Be broken with me.

I chased away the sadness and broke through tethered chains.
Found hope while fighting madness, redefining what remains.

Beautiful broken, gather up the pieces.
Much stronger rewritten. Beautiful broken.

CHAPTER 1

NO SISTER OF MINE WILL BE CARRIED OFF THE COURT

The basketball game moved at a fast pace. Our tiny high school's foul-smelling, stuffy gym was packed with screaming classmates and dozens of parents, but the tension was palpable in the air: we were at a disadvantage against the bigger team of our rival school.

But none of that mattered to me. I was just excited to be sitting on the bench, anxious to play varsity as a freshman, on the same team as my sister Kirsti, who was a junior.

McLoughlin Union High School, or Mac-Hi, as we affectionately called it, really was a small school for our even smaller town in Oregon. But we put up a fight during our sporting events and I for one was ready and anxious to show what I could do to help my fellow Mac-Hi Pioneers win.

As I was chatting with my other benched freshman teammates, I heard the familiar call of my coach yelling my last name: "Bigler!" That meant, "Hurry, take off your warmups, go sit beside me and wait to be subbed in."

The whistle blew and the adrenaline kicked in as I ran to my position, playing a shooting guard with Kirsti. Once out on the court, the echoes from the narrow rows of stands rained down on me and the rest of my team. I knew that the spectators had to look closely at the different numbers on mine and Kirsti's jerseys to tell us apart. Being the same height of about 5' 6" and with our long, light brown hair scooped up in ponytails, we looked quite a bit alike. Close up, it was easy to tell us apart, even though we both had blue eyes. Kirsti looked more like Mom with her dark blue eyes and light features while I looked more like Dad with my full lips and thick dark eyebrows.

Now that we were both out and playing together, the larger team against us wouldn't know what would hit them. Kirsti and I were both very fast and could get up and down the court at lightning speed. We were great at fast break lay-ins and stealing the ball from opponents every chance we got. Eager to show off my skills as an underclassman in front of my opponents and the gathered crowd, I launched into the fray with my teammates the second the ball entered the court.

I hadn't been in the game long before I was charging down the court, my sneakers squealing their own battle cry across the polished wood floor. My heart pumped in my chest as sweat danced along my forehead. As I moved at full speed, I turned and found myself slamming straight into a girl from the opposite team. She'd set up a screen to block me so her teammate could get by and I hadn't seen her in my blind spot.

When we made contact, it was like colliding with a brick wall. Before I knew what had happened, I was opening my eyes, trying to catch my breath with my back against the cold floor.

What just happened . . . ? I thought, blinking in confusion. *Did I pass out?* It was so hard to breathe and pain exploded throughout my head.

I tried to inhale, not knowing how much time had passed. As everything came back into focus, I noticed Kirsti's face leaning down toward mine.

She looked concerned as she asked, "You alright?"

I couldn't talk yet because I was still trying to breathe, but I was able to nod. Expecting a little sympathy from my big sis, I was surprised at the next words out of her mouth:

"Good, because no sister of mine is going to be carried off the court!"

She reached toward me and I grasped her fingers to help me up. I almost felt like I could breathe again, but my head was really hurting. Quickly, I found my parents in the crowd, halfway down the bleachers coming to check on me. I made eye contact with each of them, then forced a painful smile letting them know I was okay. They both knew how strong and sometimes stubborn I could be, but I wanted them to know I wasn't going to quit just because my head was a bit achy.

Glancing over at Coach, I realized she hadn't even got up off the bench to see if I was alright. In fact, when we made eye contact and she saw that I was up and moving again, she didn't take me out of the game either. I guess she figured I would ask to go out if I needed to, or she knew that there was no way I'd get back on the bench if I didn't have to.

Instead I got back into position and played my heart out for the rest of the quarter.

I'm glad she didn't take me out! Ever since I was small, I hated being taken out of a game. I was tough and was willing to sacrifice my body for the win. It was this instinctive drive that I couldn't resist. I'm not sure where that drive came from, but I loved being active and playing hard. I'd run through every drill until I puked, pushing myself and not cutting corners. I was always very determined to be my best.

Kirsti was always way more competitive than me, but we both played very aggressively. We were known for our smiles and happiness off the court and our viciousness once the ball was in play. I wasn't sure where we got it from, but we were fierce, making us both very unlike our big brother, who was the nicest, most laid-back guy. Nathan enjoyed sports but played more to have fun and to get in shape. He pushed himself but didn't care what others were doing around him. It wasn't until he started running marathons and lifting weights that he found that competitive side that Kirsti and I loved so much.

When the game was over, however, I began to regret pushing myself through the remaining quarters. As my adrenaline wore off and I had finished giving it everything I had like every sport I played, I soon realized my head was pounding. I was proud of myself for finishing the basketball game as a varsity player, even after getting knocked out. I knew my family doctor might not have been impressed, so I didn't let on how badly I had smacked my head. Not wanting to make another trip to see him, I didn't let any injury get in the way of finishing my season.

After I fell on my knee during one game and got a small dent in it, the doctor sent me to physical therapy. I promised to wear a knee pad, both my ankle braces and my tendon wrap around my other knee if he would let me play. I probably looked a little silly with all my preventive gear on, but I did whatever it took to keep participating. I never worried what others thought about how I looked; despite how much the other fourteen-year-old girls around me worried about their appearance, I couldn't have cared less. As long as I could play, I was happy.

Heading into spring meant softball season would begin soon, as our tiny town dusted off the snow and the green grass got ready to be manicured into a beautiful outfield. That meant it was time for me to slide headfirst into home plate and get caught in too many hotbox situations. This was one of my favorite sports because I'd started fast pitch softball when I was just eight years old in our city league. As a teenager, it was a thrill to push the limits (much to my coach's frustration).

During one game early on in the season, I was rounding second base and thought I could make it to third. Through the cheers of the crowd that met my ears as the sunshine beat down on my dusty helmet, I could hear my coach yelling at me to stay on second. Much to his dismay, however, I kept running. As I was halfway there, the third baseman caught the ball. Skidding to a half and billowing up fresh dust clouds, I started running back toward second base.

Please don't let me get tagged out, I thought as my heart hammered. *Please don't—*

But the second baseman caught the ball and groans rose amongst the people in the bleachers. I knew that if I glanced back at Coach standing on the third base line, he wouldn't be happy. Quickly, I spun once again toward third base, my eye on the ball. To my delight, it was overthrown and I dove headfirst into the hard bag. I was safe!

I stood, brushing the dirt off myself. As I looked up at Coach, I saw him shaking his head at me. At the end of the inning, I was the first one he rounded on for a lecture.

"You need to listen to me, Bigler," he snapped. "You should have stayed on second! It's too risky."

I gave him my biggest smile that usually did the trick getting me out of lots of trouble, but he didn't smile back. Both of us knew it would happen again. I thought about opening my mouth and reminding him that at least I was safe, but thought better of it. I didn't want to push it *too* far.

I remember that day was our fourth game of the season. We were on our home field at Yantis Park, where we always played our home city league games. It was located in our one and only park close to the golf course. It was unusually hot that day and the sun beat down on us, making me sweat in my white softball pants and bulky green softball jersey during warmups.

I rolled my sleeves up and tucked them under my sports bra to keep them up while I played. Even though it was hot, it was a nice change from the cool spring practices we'd been having earlier in the week. The slight wind made the heat tolerable, but I wished the uniforms were a little cooler as I stretched my socks and stirrups up over my knee and covered them with my pants.

I wasn't a fan of all the layers, but I was grateful for a little extra padding for when I would slide. Checking to see if my parents had shown up, I noticed there weren't many people there to watch us, hardly a crowd in the stands. It was normal to see mostly parents and a few of our friends from school.

I arrived early to warm up and smeared my eye black under my eyes. It was supposed to help keep the glare out of our eyes, but when I put it on, I didn't care so much what it did for me. It just made me feel tough.

After warming up, our team huddled in close with our hands in a messy pile on top of one another to say our cheer. Before our voices rang out as one, Coach looked at the entire team and said, "If Brita calls the ball, make sure to back off and let her get it!"

It was hard to hide the big grin that I wanted to release. Instead, I looked down, avoiding any eye contact with my team. I didn't like the attention he gave me, but he was right: my teammates didn't want to get in my way and at that point in the season they knew better, too. The cheer was yelled and off to the field we went.

I loved playing in the outfield. Sprinting out to center field, I was anxious for a far off ball so I could run to catch it. The first three batters made good hits and got on base, but none of the balls came close to me. Expecting a big hit from the fourth girl, I watched as she stepped up and her body shifted, knowing the ball was coming my way. It was a high pop fly and as I strained my eyes against the sun's glare, I saw the ball sail farther in than I was expecting.

I started yelling, "Mine, mine! I got it!"

I could only hope that nobody got in my way because the only thing I could see was the ball in the air. I ran at full speed, still shouting at the top of my lungs. Diving into a catch, I felt the ball connect with my mitt. Our team had its first out. Quickly, I sprang up and threw the ball to second base where the bag was tagged. That was our second out!

The crowd cheered, but somehow, amongst all the different cries of triumph and approval, I seemed to only hear my parents' voices. It was easy for me to single out their faces and shouts of encouragement that were familiar at my games. I lived for the thrill of those moments and wished they happened every hit.

After getting our third out, I jogged into the shady relief of the dugout to get ready to hit. When I was up, Coach gave me the sign to bunt. I shook my head at him. He glared at me and gave me the bunt sign again. I was fast, so he liked me to bunt, but I would much rather get a base hit any day. *What's the fun in bunting when I can swing for the fence instead?*

The chants of my fans behind the catcher washed over me like liquid courage. "Give 'em hell, Brita Gail!"

That phrase always made me giggle, but it helped me give everything I had to the game I was playing. I looked at Coach again, hoping he would give me the hit away sign, but he didn't. I sighed, grumbling under my breath as I shifted my gaze back to the pitcher. Even though I didn't want to, I reluctantly bunted the ball and flew past first base. I was safe.

Good, now I get to steal second.

As soon as the ball left the pitcher's hand for the next batter, I sprinted toward second base. This time, I slid feet first, which was rare for me.

I am safe again!

My teammate cranked the ball and hit me home, where I slid head-first, just for fun. Through the sting and the dirt, I knew I'd earned a nice new raspberry or scratch on my elbow. I loved my collection of battle wounds. The next time I was up at bat, Coach gave me the sign to "take the first pitch," which meant *don't swing.* But I had a silent rule of my own that I wouldn't break: If that first pitch was a strike, I wasn't going to sit and watch it hit the catcher's glove. This time, the pitch came and it was right in my sweet spot where I liked it: just a little high. Much to my coach's frustration, I cranked the ball right over the second baseman's head.

Safe at first, again! I am on fire today!

Coach glared at me, but forced his hands to slowly clap. I gave him another one of my signature grins and saw the hint of a smile curl at the edge of his lips. It was gone before I could be sure I even saw it.

After the game, I left the field to join my team in victory. I was a dirty, filthy mess, like I always was from sliding at as many bases as I could. My elbows and knees were proudly covered in new wounds. It was the best feeling in the world.

When chants and high fives were finished, I found my parents in the crowd. I held my elbow up so they could see. "Look, I got another one!" I declared as I showed off my new dust-covered, bleeding wound.

My mom shook her head and gave me a hug as Dad gave me a high five. We headed to the concession stand to get my favorite: a greasy ballpark burger to celebrate. I thoroughly enjoyed the calories I consumed; my activity level kept me fit and I never worried about what I put in my mouth. I spent my time playing hard, punishing my body that was always up for the challenge. Recovering from my injuries was always pretty quick and I was never down or out very long. I kept pushing myself to the physical limits that I desired, never thinking once that this body would ever let me down.

CHAPTER 2

GET OVER THE HURDLES

T rack and field was another sport I loved. At the end of my freshman year, everyone gathered out in the gorgeous weather for my favorite event: the 100-meter short hurdles. I'd had great times all season, but this was the determining day if I wanted to move forward to the state competition. I had to place first or second in this district meet or my season would be over.

Don't puke, I told myself as I took my place on the starting blocks. Every time, no matter how much I loved the race, I always got a sick feeling in my stomach. Closing my eyes, I said a silent prayer to help calm my nerves: *Dear God, please help me so I don't puke, please help me get over these hurdles and help me do my best.*

My parents were making their way to the finish line and the stands were full of cheering classmates. With my muscles stretched and my spiked sneakers grounded on the warm track, I knew I was ready. As soon as the gun fired, my feet pushed off the blocks and headed for the first hurdle, the most important hurdle to hit. I left my nervousness on the starting blocks as I sprinted forward.

I flew over each hurdle, focused only on the next one. When the last hurdle was in sight, anxiousness crept into my muscles. I was ready to be done with the race. Then I felt my foot knock against the top bar. In one heartbeat, I fell and tumbled against the hard ground.

Get up! I told myself and ignored the pain of some new bruises. *You have to finish!*

I don't know how I managed it, but within milliseconds I recovered and flew down the rest of the track. After passing the finish line, I heard my parents' screams of victory mixed with everyone else's. Glancing up, my eyes grew wide: Even though I'd fallen, I still got first place.

A tentative smile grew on my face as I caught my breath. Even though I'd gotten lucky, it wasn't over. There were still other groups, or heats, that had to run. I was bummed as I marched off the track and grabbed a bottle of cool water; that fall could have cost me going to state.

Not being disqualified was a miracle. If I would have fallen out of my lane or even stepped out of my lane at all I would have been disqualified on the spot. It was a painful wait to learn if I was fast enough to move on.

I followed my parents to the bleachers where we sat together. "You were so far ahead of those girls!" Mom exclaimed. "I can't believe you won even after falling."

We chatted and laughed, thrilled at the results of the race. I was happy to have them here cheering me on. Kirsti was at softball practice and would head over when she was done and Nathan was already at the track, hanging out with his own friends. I felt so lucky to have such a fan club.

No matter what sport I was putting my heart and soul into, my family was my biggest support. I glanced around at some of my teammates who were sitting alone on the sun-filled bleachers. Even more gratitude filled me because my parents were there with me. I knew it wasn't always easy for them to make it to all of my activities because they both worked, but somehow they made the time to be there.

Our chatter stopped when the whine of the outdoor speakers filled the air. My grip tightened around my water bottle and my throat went dry. It was time to hear the results. When the loud voice came over the intercom, I let out a cry of joy as my parents wrapped their arms around me. I was going to state! Even after falling, I had made it and I couldn't have been happier.

My parents and I traveled to Oregon State University for the big meet two weeks later. During the entire five-hour drive, I never stopped being nervous. My coach had all the stats and times for the top runners that I would be competing against. I was surprised when my coach informed me that I was third in the whole state of Oregon for the 100-meter hurdle race. My coach was pretty confident that I would place in the top two in my heat and take one of the top places in the finals.

"If you place high," Coach promised our small but talented team, "each of you will get a new pair of Nike running shoes." I grinned to myself as I watched the road go by outside the car window. I was looking forward to wearing my new shoes.

After getting settled in the hotel, my parents joined me and my team as we walked to the stadium for a short practice. We spotted a donut shop and stopped in for a snack. Every one of us packed in delicious, sugary calories, not worried one bit about the unhealthy food settling in our stomachs. Normally, my parents made sure I ate pretty healthy to keep up with my activity level, but the occasional treat wasn't a concern at all. After our donut break, we headed to the college stadium.

Even though no one was competing inside the huge open-air stadium that day, the field was full of at least a hundred people warming up and practicing. It felt good to be on the track to practice the night before the big meet. I was hopeful that my nerves would settle a little bit. Unfortunately that wasn't the case. That night in the hotel room, it wasn't easy to fall asleep.

Morning came and the competition grew near. We grabbed our gear and headed to the stadium. Not only was it packed full of competitors, but spectators as well. The butterflies in my stomach were overwhelming. Warming up with the team didn't calm my nerves either. Not long afterward, my heat was called. I hugged my parents and headed down to the starting line.

Yes, I still felt like I was going to throw up when I set my blocks on the start line, but that was normal. I wished my opponents good luck and nervously looked toward the finish line. I wanted more than anything to make it to the finals and take my place as one of the top sprinters in Oregon.

"Runners! On your mark, get set . . ." The gun sounded and I pushed off with all of my focus on the hurdle in front of me. I was surprised when my right foot was the one to go over the hurdle first.

Crap, this isn't right. I always lead with my left!

To my disappointment, my steps were off and I awkwardly made my first jump with the wrong foot. I tried to recover while keeping up my speed, but I couldn't get my steps right. Each hurdle was awkward and as I tried to make up time sprinting between hurdles, I could see people passing me. One by one, blurs of color blew by me, leaving me behind.

That one mistake cost me the entire race. Saying I was disappointed as I crossed the finish line was an understatement. Instantly, I knew I wasn't even going to make it to the finals. There wasn't another race where I could redeem myself. *It's over.*

I stepped over to my opponents and gave them high fives while I congratulated them. Little did they know that minutes ago I had been certain that they'd be congratulating me on a win. I accepted a quick hug from my opponent who would take second in state instead of me, then I slowly headed off the track. Even though I willed them to stop, tears were starting to well up in my eyes. A few slipped down my cheeks before I could stop them.

I had an inner drive to be my best. I didn't feel pressure from my parents or anyone else to try and be great; it was all a natural part of me. After all my hard work, I was furious with myself for not performing at the level I knew I could.

My parents found me quickly and I knew they could see my frustration in my flushed face. They didn't even ask about the competition. I could see tears in my mom's eyes; clearly she was hurting for me because she knew how important this was. Hugging me, she praised me for making it this far.

Dad was quiet, which wasn't normal for him. "Can you believe you made it here?" Dad began after a moment. He was doing his best to cheer me up, but in that moment I had a hard time recognizing anything except my failure.

"We are proud of you, Brita," both of my parents reminded me as we all glanced around the stadium one last time. Those words helped ease my disappointment. I realized that was a better reward than any medal I could receive.

Even without winning the state title, I continued to be a dedicated athlete. As my sophomore year began, I started getting up at five o'clock in the morning to work out at the YMCA with my friend. Then I would go home to shower quickly so I could make it to an early morning bible study class, then get to school on time.

As junior year got into full swing, I had all but forgotten my loss at the track meet my freshman year. By now, everyone at my school knew that I was the girl who was constantly going and going. I didn't like standing still. There was so much I could challenge my body to do and it always felt best when I was setting goals to make myself stronger in every sport I could put on my plate.

But one morning, something was wrong. When my alarm went off, I was too tired to get up. I'd been tired before, of course, with my busy schedule, but as I struggled to even get my head off the pillow or reach a shaky hand out toward my clock, I knew this was different. After debating with myself for a few minutes, I called my friend to cancel our early morning workout and went back to sleep a little longer. *Maybe I just need extra rest today.*

As the time came to make it to school, I still found myself weighing a million pounds. I fell asleep in all of my classes, not just the boring ones. By nighttime, I was back at home and curled in my bed without eating a thing. I was so exhausted even though I'd missed out on all of the physical activity I usually loved to do. I called my friend once more to cancel our early morning workouts for the rest of the week. It only took a few more days of worsening fatigue for me to ask my mom to get me in to see our family doctor.

After running some blood tests, it was confirmed that I had Mono, which I thought was hilarious because I sure wasn't kissing any boys. Kids at school always teased if someone got Mono; it implied that someone was kissing way too many people. I was so embarrassed and didn't want anyone to know that I had that diagnosis. I didn't have the energy to be teased about kissing people, even though everyone at school knew I wasn't the type to be kissing around. I didn't keep boyfriends long. Even though I was pursued by many guys, I was awkward around boys for some reason, getting nervous when I had a crush. It was easier for me to be friends than have serious relationships.

The fatigue had gotten so terrible that I had to stop everything I was doing. I slept constantly. My energy was zapped and I had never felt so exhausted in my life. It was terribly hard for me to be down with an illness. I wasn't used to sitting out. I did not like taking time off of sports and everything else I was doing, but I didn't have much of a choice. For two weeks I slept away nearly every hour of the day while taking medicine. When I wasn't sleeping, I was reading *Jane Eyre* or *Wuthering Heights*, writing in my journal, or watching movies. I watched *The Sound of Music*, one of my favorites, over and over.

After gathering some energy, I did my best to catch up on the homework that my friends brought me from school. Even though I didn't feel good, I was determined to keep my grades up. Recovery seemed to take forever, but I used every ounce of my minimal energy to get myself feeling better. I had faced lots of challenges so far and I wasn't going to let this defeat me.

CHAPTER 3

POLICE, A MIRACLE AND GRANDPA

When my mom answered the phone, she instantly looked upset. "Yes, this is Brita's mother . . . who is this?"

I could feel the tension building as she gripped the phone tighter and looked in my direction. Curiosity and nervousness filled me. I had a pretty good idea that it might be the police but hoped I was wrong.

I thought back to what happened on Saturday, when I was hanging out with my friends Rachel, Andrea, Katy, Seth and Matt. After chatting at my house, we had to take our friend Matt home who had an earlier curfew. The rest of us were not ready to be in for the night, so as we dropped off Matt, he said, "Hey, you guys should toilet paper my neighbor's house. He's a jerk."

We usually toilet papered people's houses that we knew, as a joke, but seeing how Rachel was always prepared for fun with toilet paper in her trunk, we decided that would be a great way to end our evening. Andrea had the getaway car parked on the street above Matt's neighbor's house. We all grabbed a couple toilet paper rolls and started hucking them up as far as we could into the large pine trees before us.

What a great yard to toilet paper! These trees are huge.

All of us laughed loudly, not caring who heard us. After we had most of the yard covered in stripes of bright white decorations, the front porch light suddenly turned on. An angry man appeared and all of us froze as a group.

"What are you doing?" he yelled. "Get out of here!"

Oh crap, run!

I began sprinting toward the getaway car, but that's when I realized that Seth wasn't with us. The rest of us piled into Andrea's car, all talking at once. As we caught our breath Andrea decided to drive quickly past Matt's house, where we spotted Seth. He clambered into the back seat, then we flew down the street back toward my house to switch cars. I thought we may have been fast enough, but from the expression on Mom's face, that idea started to crumble.

My mom's voice brought me back to the present. "That was the police station," she began with a straight face as she hung up the phone. "They want you and your friends to come in to talk to the guy you toilet papered." She held my gaze for a moment, then laughed. "I can't believe someone called the police on you."

Relief spread over me. None of us meant to cause any harm; we were just some high school kids having a little fun. When Dad got home, we told him all about it and I was even more grateful to have parents who weren't mad at me. They weren't thrilled we got caught, but they were very supportive.

I was glad to have my parents with me when we walked into that police station. After all, Dad was a lawyer and would make sure my friends and I didn't get stuck with any crime on our record.

I was having a hard time not laughing when I entered the room and looked at the faces of my accomplices. Rachel, Andrea and Katy were trying not to giggle, but Seth looked very uncomfortable. His parents were a little more strict than the rest of ours.

As we all got seated in a small space with just enough chairs for each of us, I got my first good look at Matt's neighbor. He was tall and lanky with dark brown hair and a pointy nose. He seemed very upset as he started talking as he was pointing to the lady sitting beside him: "Just so you all know, this is my friend who works with juvenile delinquents. I don't know why you children would target my house. You made a huge mess and I am very angry."

I glanced over at my dad, who confidently addressed everyone next. "I really don't think we need to involve anyone in the juvenile system. These are good kids that were just out having fun. We will make them come clean up your yard and they will not do this again."

It took a lot of convincing for Matt's neighbor to drop his plea to get a crime put on our records, but since we didn't damage anything, the police agreed if we cleaned up the mess and didn't bother the poor man again, then they would let us off free. Everyone thought it was pretty comical . . . except for Matt's neighbor and Seth's parents.

As we were leaving the police station, one of the cops stopped Seth and me. "Hey," he began with a low chuckle, "how did you guys get the toilet paper so far up in those trees? That was impressive."

I gave the cop a huge grin and ducked out of the police station with my parents laughing at my side. On the inside, I was desperately hoping I wouldn't ever have to go back to the police station for anything again.

After that incident, I did my best to stay out of trouble. Never did I think that my life would flash before my eyes when I was only seventeen. During my senior year, a friend of mine invited me on a ski trip. Dad was a great skier who taught my siblings and me how to confidently and safely make our way down the mountains near our home and I loved going fast down the steep runs. So I was thrilled when a friend of mine, Marcus and I made our way up on a gorgeous day during winter break to tear fresh tracks in the sparkling powder.

As the pale sun began to disappear behind the peaks above us, sharp cold descended and fresh snow rained down. Marcus and I made our way back to his dad's 4Runner, strapped our skis to the roof, loaded our gear and packed our shivering bodies into the car seats.

"What a blast!" I exclaimed as he pulled out onto the main mountain road. My fingers danced across the heater vent, waiting for feeling to come back into my skin.

"Yeah," Marcus agreed, his eyes on the dark road as snow billowed around us. "Thanks for coming with me."

I popped on the radio as we drove, getting just enough signal to tune in to my favorite station. Music had been a vital piece of my life so far, both playing it and listening to it and I smiled as a fun rock tune filled the chilly cab. As Marcus neared the next turn, I reached out to turn up the volume, then froze as the car's tires began to spin.

We were coming around a bend in the road, but the pavement was unexpectedly slick. Nothing in the mountain pass had been plowed or salted recently. The 4Runner needed to turn, but instead we headed straight for the edge of the cliff before us.

Oh dear God, please protect us! I prayed, clutching the edges of my seat as Marcus frantically turned the wheel to no avail. *Are we going to die here?* Everything proceeded in slow motion, in a surreal, terrifying haze. I held my breath, preparing to plummet to the bottom of the snowy mountain.

Then, for some odd reason, I thought of Grandpa. He had passed away a few years ago and maybe it was because I was so close to dying, but I remembered the day he moved on to be with God and the rest of our deceased family. Memories flooded my head, ones that played out in real time but only took milliseconds as our car careened out of control. Grandpa Walt was one of my biggest fans when I was younger. He always clapped the loudest when I practiced the piano and it had been so painful to watch him grow frail as he lost his battle with cancer.

At least I got to play for him one more time before he was gone, I thought and shut my eyes, almost hearing Grandpa's loud clap as if he were next to me then.

Suddenly, Marcus cranked the wheel to the left and the car spun in a circle on the iced road. I didn't have time to scream as we rolled over almost two times before slamming into the bank on the other side of the road. When the car came to a stop and the sounds of bent metal and broken glass fell away, an eerie silence enveloped us.

I hung upside down and sideways in the crashed vehicle, clenching my seatbelt tightly with both hands. I glanced at Marcus, my whole body shaking.

"Did that just happen?" Marcus asked quietly.

Without believing my own words, I responded, "Umm . . . yes, it did."

We both hung there in shock for a few minutes, letting reality set in. It seemed like I wasn't going to be reunited with Grandpa Walt today after all.

I noticed blood on Marcus's hand. "Are you okay?" I asked him, getting a bit panicky at the sight of his injury. "You're bleeding."

Marcus looked at his hand, then at the bit of blood that also showed up on the broken windshield where he must have cut it. "I'm fine," he insisted. "Let's get out of here."

Clumsily, I unbuckled my seatbelt and clambered out of the passenger window. Because the driver's door was smashed on the ground, Marcus climbed out of my window as well. Finding my feet on the freezing road, I saw that a huge boulder from the mountainside had smashed through the back window.

I can't believe it, I thought, saying another prayer of gratitude in my mind. *Thank you dear God that we weren't seriously injured! And that none of our other friends came with us today, or one of them could have been smashed sitting in the back seat.* I shuddered.

"Hey, look," Marcus said, pointing. "Our skis are just fine!" Somehow, they were still in one place on the roof of the 4Runner. I shook my head in disbelief, then wrapped my arms around myself in the cold. When a car came up behind us, the driver asked if we were alright. He told us to stay put and he would drive down the mountain to a phone where he could call the police and send them to us. While we waited, we clumsily dragged out our bags and extra snow gear to stay warm.

It took a while, but eventually we found ourselves in the back of a police car, trying our best to get warm as an officer began to drive us home. We hadn't been on the road long, however, before the policeman turned on his flashing lights.

"I'm sorry, guys," he said over his shoulder. "I normally wouldn't do this with people in the back, but the car in front of us right now is stolen. I need to pull them over."

Marcus and I gave each other frightened, bewildered looks. Just when we thought our death-defying evening was over, now this was going to happen?

"I've already called for backup," the officer added as he ran his siren to get the car in front of us to pull over. "You guys just sit tight while I make an arrest. Another officer will be here soon to take you the rest of the way home."

I sat shocked in the backseat, craning my neck to see out the windshield as the car in front of us slowed. When the officer got out to place the driver under arrest, I couldn't help thinking that this felt like a crazy movie. *These things just don't happen in real life,* I mused as we watched a guy get handcuffed on the hood of the car we sat in.

Luckily, the other policeman did arrive soon and we continued our journey home. Needless to say, mine and Marcus's parents were very relieved to find us unharmed except for the cut on Marcus's hand.

Grandma was there, too and she told me something I already knew: "Angels were looking out for you tonight, Brita. You were very lucky."

I nodded and gave her a hug, deciding to keep my recollections about Grandpa to myself. I knew I'd see him again, just hopefully not anytime soon.

As I wrapped up my last year of high school, I found myself anxious to take the next step in life. It was wonderful growing up in a small town with a supportive family and tight-knit community, but I was now ready to be on my own. The whole world and my future were waiting for me and I was going to meet them head on.

CHAPTER 4

THE TIME OF MY LIFE

I was more than ready for college life and had such a happy, fun outlook for my future! This was such a spontaneous and carefree part of my life with memories I would cherish long after the experiences were over. When I look back on the memories of who I was in college, I long for that girl to be with me now. The healthy, vibrant woman I loved to be with. I wish I would have nurtured my body more, not punishing it by constantly pushing it to the limits. I have looked back on this time of my life many times, so grateful I was able to do all the things I wanted. I never thought I would lose that freedom and long for those days again.

Three days after graduating high school, I left home, headed to Brigham Young University. I was so excited that I didn't want to wait until August to make the trip to Utah.

I was a mix of emotions, including being a little scared and nervous, gearing up to be away from home for more than a week for the first time in my life. Mostly, I was looking forward to staying up all night and napping during the day when I wanted, not to mention eating cold cereal for every meal (something we rarely got growing up). Let's just say I didn't have very high goals for being a grown-up.

My parents weren't able to drive with me, so I got settled in my new humble home, Cinnamon Tree Apartments, on my own. About a week later, out of the blue, Kirsti decided to come to the city of Provo with me, leaving the college she was attending in Oregon. That helped make the transition so much easier. Kirsti and I wanted to room together, so we found a small place off campus. I wasn't sad to be missing out on the dorms. Instead, it felt amazing to be independent and free. I also noticed after we'd had a chance to explore that all of the older, mature guys that lived in our complex were a nice perk as well.

Kirsti and I rode our bikes almost everywhere and shared a car that my parents got for us. Dad teased us that whoever got married last would get the car. I didn't think that I would end up with the car; I came here so I could focus on getting my elementary teaching degree. I loved children and couldn't wait to be instructing a whole room of energetic kids. Though I was focused on getting an education, I certainly wouldn't mind finding a great man to settle down with along the way. Since as long as I could remember, I'd always dreamt about being a wife and a mother.

Because of working hard, writing essays and filling out tons of paperwork, I had local scholarships that helped pay for my first year of tuition. Other than that, however, it was up to me to pay for school. My parents were always there to help financially if I was in a pinch, but mostly, I worked and went to school full-time. At times, it felt like a curse to try and manage both demanding tasks, since I had to work so hard all the time, but it was important to me that I would be graduating with hardly any debt.

I didn't always have the best luck on dates. One night, a group of us went out and were exploring. We drove up the canyon to a secluded area and got out for a hike. We came to a large fenced-in area that I wasn't familiar with.

"What is this place?" I questioned.

"It's a water tank, nothing dangerous here," my date responded, noticing my nervousness. I took a closer look at the huge water tank. It seemed like a weird place to hang out to me, but I followed along. Everyone decided it would be a good idea to jump the barbed-wire-topped fence to hang out. I was spontaneous and climbed the fence as well. *Now what?*

My date took my hand as we walked around the large weedy area that surrounded the water tank. There wasn't much to do there but talk, so it was a nice way to get to know each other, since this was our first date. After we talked and laughed for a while, we decided to head back home. As I jumped back over the fence, my wrist got caught on the barbed wire, tearing a nasty gash in my skin. Someone handed me some tissue to put on it, which helped slow down the bleeding. But after my date dropped me off at home, one of my roommates took me to the ER where I ended up needing stitches.

When the nurse came in, she gave me a stern, serious look. "I have to ask this . . ." She paused and I adjusted where I sat uncomfortably on the exam table, holding my freshly bandaged arm. *Why is she being so awkward all of a sudden?*

"What?" I innocently said.

The nurse continued, "Was this a suicide attempt?"

Surprise chilled my bones and I felt my spine straighten with shock. I was always a happy person, so a question like that, in fact, made me laugh. I understood what she meant because of the location of the injury, but to me it was just silly.

"No!" I almost shouted. "This was not a suicide attempt. I was climbing over a fence and caught my arm on some barbed wire." It was embarrassing having to defend myself from something so far from myself that I had never even thought about. I had never been accused of something so serious and it made me wonder how many people this woman had stitched up that were trying to take their lives.

Those thoughts saddened me. I was so glad that I wasn't in that mental state myself and I was sure that I wouldn't ever have to go through something like that with anyone in my family. I was so blessed and, once again, I said a silent prayer to thank God for His protection and for my happiness. The nurse seemed content with my answer and finished stitching up my wrist.

The whole situation made me cherish my life and I wrote my second song that semester. Of course, it was inspired by all of the dating I was enjoying and I couldn't help but dream about my happily ever after that I hoped I would eventually find. Dating was a little turbulent as I seemed to fall hard for the guys I liked. It wasn't always easy letting go or breaking up, even if I was the one ending it.

The song I wrote was called "Only Time Can Tell." One of the lines included my hopes for a relationship that I longed for.

"In his eyes I see the rising sun. Deep inside I hope that he's the one.

Only time can tell how things will be. All that I can do is wait and see."

I was anxious to find my happily ever after and found myself daydreaming about my future when I should have been studying.

My brother Nathan ended up moving to Utah, too, during my second year. My siblings and I had a blast experiencing college together. We spent a lot of time biking, hiking, going to the gym to work out, running and rollerblading together. Academically, however, my sophomore year started getting a lot harder for me. I had always been a good student, but I was starting to struggle to retain information in some of my classes. Not thinking much of it, I found cute guys to be my tutors to get me through. I did think it was weird that simple classes were not making sense, but I thought perhaps it was just the stress of a busy college life. Plus, I wasn't always getting much sleep, staying up late visiting with friends, getting up early to go to class, working and dating. I was also dealing with daily headaches and frequent migraines.

But there wasn't much that could keep me down. I merely learned how to deal with the headaches and push through. Most people had no idea that I was in pain all the time because my smile still shone strongly.

When telemarketing started to get old, I decided I needed a change of scenery and went looking for a landscaping job. I craved an active, physical job where I wasn't stuck sitting around my whole shift. I was ready to lay sod, mow lawns, dig ditches, or any other hard labor that might come up. When I arrived at the address from an advertisement I'd seen, I thought I had to be in the wrong place. It didn't look like a typical landscaping gig: the mansion in front of me with a huge yard was a little intimidating.

I pushed the button on the back service gate and announced that I was there for an interview. To my surprise, I was welcomed by an amazing yard crew that took care of the beautiful house and yard. I spent the next two years working there. It was a job that I loved: not only did we deadhead flowers and pick weeds, but we also cleaned cars and the inside of the mansion.

The worst job I had there was stringing miles of Christmas lights during the holidays on all of the many trees in the enormous yard. Other than getting sick of untangling lights, wrapping and unwrapping trees, I loved being out of an office and outside most of the time.

While getting through my general ed classes, I had decided to start out as an Elementary Teaching major. Kids were always a favorite of mine. I only had to fill in as a substitute for elementary school twice, however, before realizing that being a teacher was not the career for me. I still loved and adored children, but just knew I was not cut out to be a teacher.

So I switched to an English major next, since I have always loved to write and had dreamt of being an author. As a kid, I had many notebooks full of half-finished stories that showcased my vivid imagination. But after I started taking more English classes, I wasn't falling in love with it, either. Believe it or not, there was too much writing! And I wasn't interested in writing what the professors wanted me to write.

I decided to experiment again. I dabbled in dance classes and art and loved those creative environments. One day, a friend of mine who knew I was taking art classes came into my apartment and told me I should check out a brand new major. It was the first year BYU offered Computer Animation and as soon as I met the professor and saw the syllabus, I knew that's what I wanted to do.

Even though I could hardly turn on a computer at that point in my life, I instantly changed my degree to Industrial Design with an emphasis in animation. Learning new talents and using my artistic background, I thrived in my new major.

Because computer animation was new, we had to take quite a variety of classes. At one point, we made molds of frisbees and screwdrivers; then I found myself in lots of drawing classes, a computer programming class and a welding class.

Welding was interesting, especially one particular moment: While using a spot welder, a spark got in my hair and caught it on fire. I was thankful for the guy who ran across the room, yelling, "Your hair's on fire!" I had no idea he was talking about me until he started pounding the top of my head to put the fire out. It was then I could smell burnt hair. I panicked, fearing I'd lost half of my hair. Thankfully, after close inspection, I found that I had only lost the top layer of my thick hair. It wasn't noticeable to anyone but me after I cut off the singed ends that were left. Funny luck again.

It was a learn-as-you-go major and because it was new, there was a lot of trial and error with my classes. We learned new programs and didn't have a lot of help in troubleshooting.

Our homework usually consisted of going to watch the newest movie that was out with good effects or the newest animation. It was the perfect major for me to pursue because it didn't feel like work at all. There were only three girls in my major, which I didn't mind; it was great being around a bunch of guys. I was still single, after all!

With the computer skills I learned along with my natural talents, abilities and passion, I ended up getting a job doing graphic design. My junior year of college, I said goodbye to landscaping and started working for a fast-paced magazine company. I worked long hours, trying to keep up with the demand of the magazine. I wouldn't realize until a few years later how much that stress wreaked havoc on my body.

CHAPTER 5

NOT ANOTHER BLIND DATE

I had a list of rules when it came to my future husband. Being so social during college, I dated lots of boys, sometimes a different one at each meal, so I had my personal standards set clearly. But I wasn't having much luck in the *serious relationship* department.

There was Ryan, the cocky pilot whom I liked but my family detested. He was fearless, confident and knew what he liked. Even though some of his comments were superficial and rude, he always followed them up with the nicest things that I wanted to hear. But about six months into our relationship, I woke from a dark fog, realizing the emotional abuse I had been enduring. Though it was a hard one to end, it was a relief to say goodbye to Ryan.

Toward the end of my college career, there was Josh. He was a few years older than me and was a pretty strong magnet for my heart. We both loved to play the guitar and sing and when our voices harmonized together on Sunday evenings, it was magical. We'd been dating on and off for years and back when I was nineteen, I even thought he would propose. His family loved me and I loved them, but Josh couldn't shake the idea that there might be someone *better* for him out there in the world.

That's why, after all the heartbreak I had endured, I wasn't excited to go on yet another blind date. My good friend Sandi wanted to set me up. Since I loved her, I agreed to go to a movie with her husband's friend, Jeff. Sandi, her husband and I went to pick up Jeff one evening at his house.

His smile was the first thing I noticed. *He is kind of cute, but I'm done with boys.* Right away, I saw that Jeff was cute and had gorgeous hazel eyes, making me a little more interested in this date.

He shook my hand as he entered the car. We didn't talk much as we headed to the movie theater. The tension was palpable and awkward. Then, in the middle of the movie, Jeff answered his phone. I stared in shock as he had a full conversation during our date as the big screen's light flashed around us. He didn't even get up to leave to take the call.

He is so immature! I can't believe I'm on a date with this guy!

The movie couldn't have ended sooner. Instead of Sandi and Rick taking me back to my apartment, they took me to Jeff's house, suggesting Jeff take me home himself. I sent Sandi an irritated scowl. She smiled as she and her husband dropped us off at Jeff's house, where he needed to get his keys and then take me home. We walked into his family's log house where, at the age of twenty-one, he still *lived with his parents*.

Being forward, I asked, "So, who were you talking to during the movie?"

Jeff looked at me awkwardly. "Oh, sorry about that. It was one of my friends who I haven't seen in a long time. I have been trying to get a hold of him."

Okay, so at least he wasn't talking to another girl.

As we entered his family room, I looked up and saw a number of stuffed animal heads on the wall. "So, does your dad like to hunt?" I asked sarcastically.

Jeff laughed. He told me the condensed version of how his dad got each taxidermy trophy. I suddenly started feeling more at ease. That kind of conversation was familiar and easy for me as my dad hunted, too.

As he spoke, I glanced over and suddenly noticed how Jeff's beautiful eyes sparkled with the humor of his current tale. I found myself laughing and enjoying being around him so much that I even agreed to another date. I was pleasantly surprised, especially since the night hadn't started out so well.

As we talked, getting to know each other, we discovered we both loved sports. Not just "Oh yeah, they're cool to watch from time to time" but "I'm a huge, raving fan and participant of whatever-I-can-get-my-hands-on sports fanatic!" That was so refreshing and I think I surprised him because he hadn't met a lot of girls like me in that arena. We also discovered that we both enjoyed the outdoors, our families and so much more.

It was a little weird but fantastic to discover as the night wore on that we had similar goals and dreams, too. It made me a little nervous, but in a good way, to feel such an immediate connection with someone. And by the end of our long conversation that night, the cuteness that I noticed when I met Jeff turned into a breathtaking attraction.

I certainly had not expected to hit it off with my blind date, especially an immature guy who talked on his phone in movie theatres. Yet there I was, completely intrigued. Before he took me home, Jeff gave me a warm hug. As he went in for a kiss, I found myself letting him. And I found myself thinking about his luscious, soft lips long after he took me home.

From that day forward, we found ourselves together, going on hikes, hanging out with friends, or just having relaxing conversations. My heart, however, wasn't ready to fully open up again. I wasn't prepared that he was suddenly just my type.

Jeff was further along than I was in our relationship, ready to commit to being exclusive after two weeks of casually dating. I don't think his heart had been warped like mine from past partners. I was a little gun-shy and told him I still wanted to date other people. As I told him the news, Jeff was disappointed and his trusting smile disappeared. I felt bad hurting him, but I just couldn't commit to someone so fast. So I kept going on dates with other guys when I wasn't spending time with Jeff. But when I was out with them, I found myself thinking about Jeff, which was a new experience for me. Usually I wouldn't think twice about another guy while I was out with someone else.

It caught me off guard how much I was thinking about Jeff. It didn't take long for me to realize I was ready to give him a shot. Not just dating for an extended period—I could actually try a committed relationship. It was clear that I was falling hard for him . . . and fast. So, one afternoon in July, I called Jeff to invite him to lunch. Flurries of excitement raced through my stomach as I checked my hair and simple makeup in the mirror one more time before stepping outside. I was ready to date exclusively and couldn't wait to tell Jeff I now felt the same way he did.

He surprised me by saying, "Actually, you were right. I think we should date other people."

To say I was shocked was putting it lightly. Dejected and embarrassed, I was sure that I had lost him. The second he went on a date with another girl, he would forget all about me. I knew right then that I would always regret losing him. When I got home that night, I prayed that it wouldn't take him long to realize I was the one that he wanted. After all, I didn't know how much I liked him until I thought I lost him forever.

Luckily, after going on only one date, Jeff decided he wanted to be exclusive, too. One of the things I loved about this man was his sincere feelings. We went on to date exclusively for just a month before Jeff turned to me one evening as we walked in the park, looked into my eyes and said, "I love you."

Honestly, it kind of freaked me out. My walls were still up emotionally and it was going to take a lot to break them down. I loved the way he said it anyway, despite how I didn't say "I love you" back for quite a while. But the cool thing about Jeff was it didn't matter to him if I said it back.

Genuine love gushed out of this gentleman. He was so thoughtful, happy, funny and sweet. I thought about the guys I had dated before him and I realized that he was so different, so kind, sincere and dedicated to the point that it was often the opposite of what I had encountered in the past. There was no stringing me along, nor was he looking for someone better to come along. He knew what a catch I was and it felt good. And I felt the same way about him.

That's when I found myself falling in love with Jeff. He was so caring about my needs, always making sure I was warm enough on our frequent evening strolls. Best of all, he encouraged me to be me. He didn't want me to try and be like someone else. He got my sarcastic humor and I got his, so we laughed a lot at ourselves and each other. Jeff always had his arm around me or was holding my hand. My walls melted away very quickly and I found myself trusting him with all my heart.

One special night, three months after we started dating, Jeff took me to Rock Canyon, a beautiful park just outside Provo where we hiked together often. I kept glancing over at him because his behavior was kind of odd that evening. He was usually so calm and laid back, but he was talking fast and kept looking around like he lost something. As we headed up one of the usual trails, I brushed it off, choosing to enjoy the serene air around us.

As Jeff pulled me up onto the huge rock that we liked to rest at, I was surprised when Jeff suddenly dropped to one knee on the hard surface. I felt tears spilling down my cheeks, but there was no hesitation when I burst out an enthusiastic, "YES!"

I couldn't believe we were on the same page and that we were both completely in love with each other. I felt so safe in his arms, but I couldn't ignore the irony of how I'd ended up falling for someone who went against all the rules I had set for myself. Here's that list I mentioned at the start of the chapter and how Jeff defied all of my expectations:

1. I wouldn't marry someone who still lived at home.
   a. He was living at home when I met him.
2. I wouldn't marry someone I met on a blind date.
   a. I went on too many bad ones to have hope it could possibly ever work!
3. I wouldn't marry someone younger than me.
   a. Jeff is a year younger than me.
4. I wouldn't marry someone right off his church mission.
   a. He had only been off his mission for two months when I met him.
5. I would date someone *at least* one full year before I would even consider marriage.
   a. We met in June, got engaged in August and were married that December.
6. I wouldn't marry someone from Utah.
   a. Except for his two-year church mission, he had lived in Utah his whole life.

The list went on, but I happily threw that list away and married Jeff!
Best. Decision. Ever.

There were so many things in my life that I wasn't sure of, but one decision I was very sure of was marrying Jeff. I had never believed it when people said things like, "I just knew that he was the *one*." That sounded so silly to me. But with Jeff, I suddenly knew exactly what they meant; I had found my happily ever after.

I thought I had been in love before, but with Jeff, I experienced something entirely new: it felt like an invisible force grounding me, powerful but as subtle as gravity. I had never felt so safe or loved in such a short amount of time. And these feelings between us were so strong, fun and effortless every day. I somehow knew that this man would be there for me through anything. I could see it in his sweet actions, hear it in the sincerity of his voice and feel it in his soft love that pulled me to him like a strong magnet.

In some of our many conversations, Jeff and I talked about how we both wanted a big family: six to eight kids at least. I had always wanted a big family and I was thrilled that Jeff did as well. We also dreamed about adopting kids one day and the possibility of being foster parents. We both agreed that we would build our family as we felt inspired by God, hoping to be blessed with a house full of children.

I knew that I didn't want to wait too long to start having babies; I wanted them close together and to have lots of them. Our future looked so bright. Our dreams were big and our love was so strong. Little did I know that our great love was about to be tested.

CHAPTER 6

I SHOULD BE GLOWING

Not long after being home from our honeymoon, Jeff's dad showed us an old farm house that he owned, that used to be Jeff's great-grandmother's. He asked us if we would like to buy it. Even though it was a major fixer-upper, when I walked through the house, I fell in love with it. My fixer-upper vision was very strong and I could imagine this neglected house that was trashed by renters turning into my simple, dream farmhouse with some love, a lot of hard work and more money than we had planned on.

Not only were Jeff and I working long hours and Jeff was also attending school, but we started renovating our house, while renting an apartment from Jeff's parents. We had to basically gut it, put new carpet in, take down walls and ceilings and it became much more work than we had anticipated. After having to get new sheetrock in our living room, we came over to check on things and the sheetrock was all wet. A huge unexpected expense came up when that led to us replacing the roof.

Instead of finishing the house before we moved in, our budget was spent and we got the bare minimum done so we could settle into living in a construction zone. It was not easy to live in the chaos. My brother, Nathan, spent a lot of time helping us fix up the house, which was good because he actually knew what he was doing. Jeff and I were hard workers, but we didn't always know how to do things the right way. We teased that everything we did was "good enough;" neither of us were perfectionists.

My dream home that we thought we'd have done in three weeks was turning into a money pit and taking forever to get done. At least we had one working bathroom, a place to sleep and the kitchen was somewhat functional. And the acre of land that came along with our house gave us the country feel we both loved.

Amidst the chaos of working long hours and fixing up our house, I started wondering when we should start planning our family. It didn't take long for a pregnancy test to be positive and I was ecstatic in preparing to be a mom, the one thing I truly wanted to be.

As much as I was looking forward to being a mom, pregnancy wasn't too kind to me.

Where is this "glow" that everyone is always talking about? I was excited, but I surely did not have the "glow" as I was too busy throwing up in the morning, noon and at night as well.

Perhaps the worst thing was how everyone loved to share their unsolicited advice by telling me, "Don't worry, the morning sickness goes away after the first trimester." I know they were trying to give me a thread of hope that it would soon be over.

They were wrong.

Continuing after the first trimester, I was still very sick all day long.

Even though I didn't feel great, I was delighted to go to my ultrasound appointment to find out the gender of our first baby. Jeff and I were so excited and had talked about it for weeks. We had many conversations like the one we had in the car on the way to the appointment that day. "So," Jeff smiled as he asked, "Do you think we are having a boy or girl?"

I rubbed my hand on my belly as I spoke. "I always thought I would have a boy first, so I'm pretty sure this is going to be a boy." Because my oldest sibling was a wonderful big brother, the thought of having a boy first seemed natural to me.

"Yes, I think you are right . . ." Jeff started, then quickly added, "Well, I don't know . . . it could be a girl." We both laughed, knowing that we didn't have a clue what was in store for us and couldn't wait for our gender reveal! We didn't care if the baby was a boy or girl, but we were so happy to know which one we were having so we could start buying cute little clothes!

The friendly nurse smiled at us. "Do you want to know the gender of your baby today?" She said this as she rubbed cold gel on my stomach with the ultrasound wand.

"Yes!" I nearly yelled in anticipation.

"Looks like you are having a little girl."

Happy tears rolled down my face as I took in the news. I couldn't wait to hold my perfect little girl in my arms. This ultrasound made everything seem more real. We had already decided if this baby was a girl, we would name her Landan. I longed to bask in this happiness, but as the ultrasound continued on, however, we were worried there might be complications. The look on the nurse's face made us a little nervous. Our concerns were verified when she left and sent the doctor in to talk to us.

"How exciting, you guys are having a girl," the doctor said dryly as he was looking down at my chart.

As I listened to him intently, the doctor didn't sound excited. I could see by the twitch of his hands and how he kept clearing his throat that he didn't have all great news. My stomach started to flutter as I braced myself.

"So, I am a little concerned about something we found on the ultrasound." I held my breath, concerned for my precious baby. Without even thinking about it, Jeff grabbed my hand and we looked at each other nervously. My heart was racing. "This condition happens in about one percent of pregnancies," the doctor continued. "The baby has a two-vessel umbilical cord."

That meant nothing to me. My face was blank and so was Jeff's. "So what does that mean?" I asked quickly, fearing the worst.

"Basically, with this kind of abnormality," the doctor continued, "your baby has a high risk for problems with her heart and kidneys and . . . she has a high chance of being Down Syndrome. Preterm labor and other complications can also put your baby at high risk."

The doctor and the nurse went on to explain that because now it was considered a high-risk pregnancy, I had to have ultrasounds regularly and meet with a specialist nearly as frequently. It was a very stressful time for us. I worried about my baby's health. When Jeff came home from a long day's work, I could see it etched in his face, too.

Not only was I so stressed about the baby news, my job was becoming more and more unstable. After watching the company fire my friend, who was an amazing graphic designer, the year before, putting me in charge, I started getting nervous about my job. I was being paid pretty well, but the boss's wife, Penny, didn't like me for some reason and kept confronting me about the time I was putting into the magazine.

Even though I worked constantly for them, putting in ridiculous hours and always meeting the insane deadlines that were set for me, Penny wasn't satisfied. It was a very frustrating time for me, since not only was I sick from my pregnancy and worried about my baby, but also the stress of the job was too much. I was such an honest, hardworking employee and couldn't handle the negative comments I was getting from Penny and other employees, who kept acting like my job was in jeopardy.

Quickly, rumors were flying around the office and I started looking for other jobs, just in case. I wasn't that surprised when Penny showed up at my house one afternoon to fire me. I was so angry because I never did anything wrong and put in so much time and effort into the job. Hearing the lies Penny told about me from coworkers back at the office was even more infuriating.

I'm not one to sit back and be attacked so I didn't have the nicest things to say back at her. I was hurt since I had put so much time and effort trying to do the best I could for the company. Not long after I was let go, the company went bankrupt and shut down. It was clear to me that poor management was actually the source of their troubles, not me. Nonetheless, all of the stress was hard on my body. I was irritable and didn't quite feel like myself, but blamed it on pregnancy hormones.

The funny thing was, even though Penny fired me, I got a glowing recommendation from my boss (Penny's husband) for a new design position at a new company. He always treated me well and knew the kind of employee I was. It was a very stressful time because the job Jeff was working at went out of business the same week I lost my job. We were not having the best of luck.

It only took me a few weeks of unemployment to start my new job with my growing belly. The new company was easy to work with and it wasn't long before they knew what an asset I was to their company. They were very forward about how much they appreciated me and loved my work. After proving myself, soon I was working from home creating computer fonts for them. It was perfect timing since Jeff and I would be leaving soon for our first summer sales adventure.

Jeff was selling pest control to support him in school the other seasons of the year, so we moved to California for the summer. I worked in the sales office, scheduling appointments and other things while I awaited the arrival of our sweet girl, while I created the computer fonts for my other job after working all day. Even though I didn't feel good, I was used to pushing through hard things and getting things done. It wasn't always easy, but I made it work. I never made excuses for myself, I just rested when I could, threw up often while at work and somehow just got through it.

Because I had a high-risk pregnancy, I was nervous to move to a different state for treatment, but loved my new OB immediately. He assured me that he was familiar with my baby's condition and kept a close watch on us.

My free time was spent in the pool or the ocean, which felt so good on my aching, expanding body. As I was floating in the waves, I opened my heart up for whatever God had in store for us. Jeff and I discussed that we would love this little girl no matter how she came. I made that promise to myself and to her, as I floated on the water and she floated inside of me.

"It's going to be okay," I whispered to her over and over.

Even though I continued to throw up my entire pregnancy, I continued to work. My parents came into town just in time for me to go into labor. Relief washed over me as we welcomed a healthy baby girl in July 2004, with no complications or health concerns and no Down Syndrome! Tears rolled down both my and my husband's cheeks as we held this beautiful little sweetheart and we named her Landan.

Landan was the cutest little baby; she had bright blue eyes and wispy little bits of light brown hair. Her lips were full and she had the cutest little nose. Her short little upper body was followed by long gangly legs. I thought she was the most beautiful baby I had ever seen.

My dad had to get back to work after a few days, but Mom was able to stay with us for a week as we adjusted to new life with a baby. It was so nice to have the help and I was so grateful that my parents were always so willing to be there for us. Some of Jeff's family had come to visit us in California before Landan was born since a few of his siblings ran a marathon there. We went to the zoo, the beach and supported the marathoners and it was so nice to be with them there for a visit. We moved back to Utah just three weeks after Landan was born, stopping in Oregon to see my parents on the way through. Jeff's family was excited to meet our new little bundle. It was a crazy time. I enjoyed being a mother just like other new moms I knew, but it was hard having a newborn. I was exhausted. The trip was extra long, as we took lots of breaks to hold and feed Landan along the way.

Breastfeeding wasn't going so well for any of us and after pumping for breast milk and using formula to help supplement my minimal supply of milk, eventually we got into a routine. All of us were able to get past the every-hour cries and get more rest. Even in the middle of the night, I would take precious moments after Landan fell asleep to brush the cheek of my little miracle. I would linger in the rocking chair, not wanting to put her back to bed, knowing she would stay safe in my arms. My heart could not have been more full with the love I had for her.

Being pregnant had not brought out the best in me. From week two to forty, I just didn't feel like myself. I angered easily and was grumpy a lot, complaining and frowning constantly at how unlike me I felt. Brushing off the heaviness, I attributed everything to hormones and work stress, trying to assure myself that all of the negative feelings were temporary and I would be back to myself in no time.

Jeff constantly hugged me and reassured me, saying things like, "You have been so sick the entire pregnancy and all those extra hormones can't make you feel good. You feel terrible all the time. That would make me grumpy too." He had been so patient with me when I hadn't been patient with myself.

After working hard to get back to my pre-pregnancy weight, happily, it didn't take long for me to become pregnant again. My sweet husband and I were excited to be getting ready for baby number two and for Landan to have a little brother or sister to play with. I had always wanted to have kids close together so I was thrilled. I felt so blessed that God was sending me another baby especially when I knew plenty of people that couldn't get pregnant. Although I was so sad for the friends who were struggling, I couldn't contain my happiness.

Of course, we announced our pregnancy as soon as we found out, because of our excitement. The only negative part was when my throwing up started and terrible headaches were triggered. They weren't fun, but everything seemed pretty normal until I sadly miscarried in December 2004, when Landan was just five months old.

After calling the doctor's office to get advice about the miscarriage, I went upstairs to my room to sob. For the next several days, I grieved deeply for the loss of our unborn child.

It's amazing how connected I had been to the newly formed baby that had been developing inside me. Because I was only around twelve weeks along, I didn't feel like I got much support from those around me to deal with my loss. Somehow since I wasn't further along, I was just supposed to get over it. I was reminded that I didn't get to hold the baby, so it really wasn't a loss, which couldn't have been further from the truth. Nobody really knew how hard I was grieving, except Jeff, who was grieving by my side. His strong but tender heart was breaking right along with mine.

Then out of the darkness, a small light flickered. Three hard months after the miscarriage, we discovered we were pregnant again. After having a miscarriage, I was nervous about announcing another pregnancy and worried every day over the baby. Time seemed to take forever getting to my twenty-week ultrasound. I held my breath as the same cold wand was rubbed around on my belly, hoping for a healthy baby. We were thrilled to find out we would soon be parents to another girl. I hoped that Landan and her sister would become as close as my sister and I were.

That summer we lived in Kent, Washington, for Jeff's seasonal sales work. I didn't love living in a place with so much rain and clouds—it was so different from anywhere I had ever lived, even though I grew up in Oregon. I tried to blame it on the gloomy skies, but I seemed to be dealing with some depression during this pregnancy, depression that I couldn't quite admit. I had so much to be grateful for, after all. I couldn't be depressed.

It didn't help that I was experiencing even worse headaches this pregnancy. I couldn't explain it. It was as if my body didn't like being pregnant. Luckily, we made some good friends and as much as we could, enjoyed being in Washington, clouds and all. I have to admit I was thrilled to return to our old country home in very sunny Utah at the end of the summer and I carried the baby until her birth, about a month after Christmas. She had a full head of dark brown hair and, after a traumatic birth, was a bit swollen and bruised. Slowly her bruising and swelling calmed down and her blue eyes sparkled. She was such a pretty baby.

We had a hard time naming her, but with the pressure of having to leave the hospital soon, Jeff and I got out our list and finally made a decision. We named her Taylor and it seemed to fit her just right.

Once home, as I looked in the mirror, I knew I looked pretty good for a momma with three pregnancies and two little girls. However, I knew I could look better and I especially wanted to *feel* better. I'd done it before. To lose my pregnancy weight this time, I trained for a half marathon. It was hard work, especially since I had always been a sprinter, not a long-distance runner. I trained with a dear friend of mine and it was so fun being with her and working towards such a huge goal together. I felt alive and free, even as I pushed the double jogging stroller in front of me nearly every day. My muscles remembered strength and speed, but not always endurance. That took some time to build up.

I still feel bad for the people that saw me puke just before reaching the finish line, the poor folks who were waiting to cheer on their loved ones. Still, as I crossed the finish line to the applause of my little family, I was so proud to have finished such a great accomplishment. Getting back to my pre-pregnancy weight was nice, too. My adrenaline had hardly faded when I began to plan my next half marathon.

Not only was I finding time to run, I continued to work from home, making computer fonts for the same company. They were a great company to work for and, being able to set my own hours, it was a mother's dream. I had a great job while I stayed home raising my kids. I picked up more work doing other freelance graphic design jobs. I always had as much work as I wanted—and for us, that was just enough to have some extra spending money.

Usually, we used any extra money to dump into our old fixer-upper house, which reminded me of the home my parents remodeled when I was young. My parents had taught me to work hard and I loved the feeling of accomplishment as we fixed up our own house. Jeff and I had done lots of remodeling over the years and did most of the work by ourselves, although we got lots of help with drywall and framing walls from my brother, Nathan. It felt like we were constantly working on a project and were so glad to have his help.

I always had plenty to do while the girls were taking their naps, or after they went to bed at night. The old dresser we bought at the thrift store that we turned into our kitchen island was one of my favorite projects. The finishing touches were what I loved, painting and adding that new layer of design, seeing all of the hard work come together to create something new and beautiful. As I had been all my life, I thrived being busy. I was joyful and I managed my time well to get everything done, especially spending quality time with my girls, which was most important to me. The girls were getting so big. I loved putting Landan's light brown hair up into little pigtails and Taylor's hair had turned from dark brown at birth into a light blonde, which made her eyes stand out even more. I was living my dream life and couldn't be happier, but every now and again, there was a heaviness that crept in that I couldn't quite describe.

CHAPTER 7

SANDWICH

After my race, I felt unstoppable. It was the first time in a couple of years that I actually felt good emotionally and physically. Then, about ten months after Taylor was born, I discovered I was pregnant again with our third baby. Jeff and I were thrilled! Unfortunately, I was terribly sick all over again for months on end. Even though my stomach was always twisted with nausea, I couldn't be happier to keep building the family I had always wanted. All I had to do was look at my beautiful munchkins to know that it was well worth it.

It was the beginning of summer, but one afternoon when the weather wasn't terribly hot and filled with warm sunshine, Jeff and I got the girls ready to go to the park. It was important to both of us to spend extra time with them before the next baby came. We lived on a small farm, with a busy road in front of our house, so we had to drive two minutes away to our favorite park.

Even though I still wasn't feeling well at eight months pregnant, I did my best to keep up with Jeff and the kids, pushing them on the swings, chasing them happily in circles and going down the slides with them. We were rarely the kind of parents who sat on the sidelines watching them play. We enjoyed being a part of their lives. I was pushing Taylor on the swing when Jeff and Landan came over.

"Are you ready to go?" Jeff asked with a smile.

As I looked at Jeff, my brain tried to say, "Yes, let's go." But for some reason what came out of my mouth instead was, "Sandwich."

I froze, confusion and panic flooding my mind. My hands missed the swing the next time Taylor came toward me as my mouth went dry. *What just happened . . . ?*

Jeff laughed at my odd response and I assumed he thought I was teasing him. He probably just thought I was hungry, but it didn't take him long to notice the panic in my eyes. I tried to speak another time, but again, something weird came out, nowhere near the fear I was trying to convey. What was wrong with me?

Apparently crying must not take very much brain power, because even though I wasn't able to form the words I wanted, the tears still knew how to fall. I pointed to my brain and shook my head as worry blossomed on my husband's face.

"Here, sit down," Jeff said as he gently placed his hand on my back to steady me.

I sat slowly on one of the park benches as the girls continued to play.

"Are you okay?" Jeff asked.

I shrugged my shoulders hopelessly. Every part of me wanted to talk, but my brain wasn't able to process words. I slumped forward in defeated silence. Jeff hurried and scooped up Taylor from the swing, herded Landan and steadied me with his free hand to get me to the car. As I silently relaxed in the hot car, I was very scared. I had never experienced something like this and I feared something could be very wrong. I lovingly touched my growing belly and hoped the baby and I would be okay.

Jeff immediately called my doctor to tell him what was going on. The doctor didn't seem too concerned, but was able to get me into his office the next day. After about an hour, the episode had run its course, all the numbness went away and my speech was back to normal. Jeff and I were very frightened and concerned for my health, but we were getting so close to my due date. Above all, we were more concerned for the health of the baby.

"Well, Brita," my doctor began after running some tests, "this looks like just a weird anomaly. Since it hasn't happened before, I believe it's something that's been triggered by your pregnancy. But please call me if it happens again."

I sighed, not entirely happy with such a vague, unhelpful answer. Even though it had been an odd and scary experience, I decided to mirror my doctor and not be too worried. We hoped another episode wouldn't happen again.

Once again, I delivered a healthy baby that fall; this time, it was a boy we named Callen. He had the cutest squeaky little cry. Because he only had long, wispy bits of hair on the sides of his head, we teased that he had grandpa hair. He was such a cute little guy. Landan and Taylor were thrilled to be big sisters. Even though they were just three and one and a half years old, they were such good helpers as soon as Callen and I got home from the hospital. They got me diapers and helped in any way they could. Luckily, I didn't have any more trouble being able to speak the words that I wanted. We just blamed the episode at the park on the pregnancy and didn't think much more of it.

That was, until I got pregnant again.

CHAPTER 8

AM I PREGNANT AGAIN?

G etting into a schedule with another newborn took some time. It was such a joy having a little boy join our family and Landan and Taylor were the best little helpers. They were so excited to have a baby brother and I felt like I spent my entire day putting Callen back and forth on Landan and Taylor's laps. It was so cute and I loved my sweet little people. I felt so blessed to have three healthy children and I loved being a mom.

Six months later, I was still trying my best to create a "normal" schedule with a baby and two toddlers. Despite the new coordination and sleeplessness, I still felt immensely blessed by my helpful little girls and the new addition to our family. One Saturday, I stood in the laundry room while Callen was napping, taking the moment of relative quiet to catch up on folding tiny pairs of pants. Landan and Taylor were nearby, chatting with me while I worked.

Suddenly, black spots started floating in and out of my eyesight. When I glanced at the kids, I saw confusion on their little faces. I realized the words I was thinking weren't the words that were coming out of my mouth.

Frustrated tears formed in my eyes. *Why is this happening again?* Panic boiled inside my gut when I couldn't make coherent sentences. All of a sudden, my lips and tongue went numb, as well as my right hand and foot. I limped to the other side of the house, searching desperately for Jeff as my mind tried to process what was going on.

Wait . . . This has happened before and last time . . . Oh my gosh, am I pregnant again?!

I couldn't process that thought, nor could I voice it to Jeff when I found him in the living room. When his eyes met mine, all I could do was stare at him and hope he would know that our greatest fear came true: it was happening again.

Jeff helped me into bed. As the kids played, he sat by me as the episode ran its course. It lasted for thirty minutes, full of an eerily familiar sense that

I didn't like at all. Exhaustion hit me once I was able to find my voice again and I knew I wasn't getting up the rest of the day.

With Jeff by my side, I was finally able to speak: "Jeff, this is the same thing that happened when I was pregnant with Callen. So I think I might be pregnant again."

Although that wasn't the way I wanted to find out that we were expecting once more, after confirming with a pregnancy test, Jeff and I celebrated the anticipation of another child. After a quick look at my calendar, I calculated that I was only about six weeks along. With Callen, my episode had occurred in my final month of pregnancy, but now, so early on, I'd already had one.

Does this mean I am going to have this problem during this whole pregnancy? How am I going to take care of the three kids I already have?

My OB encouraged me to go to a neurologist, so I met with Dr. Vincent, a specialist, to have an EEG. The results showed that I was having seizures, but it was unclear if the seizures were the reason I couldn't form the correct words and felt that numbness. When Dr. Vincent finally shared this truth with us, Jeff and I stared at one another. The doctor suggested I could take seizure medication to try and stop the episodes. But as my hand went down to touch my stomach, I wasn't so sure if that was the best idea.

As Jeff and I talked about the pros and cons of such a medication on the way home, I decided that since the seizures were not severe, I would not take any drugs while I was expecting. I didn't want the side effects of the medicine to harm my baby, who wasn't due for several months still.

I was determined to make the best of these seizures, no matter how frightening and debilitating they were. With the same drive I used when I was facing an opponent on the basketball court or on the softball pitch as a teenager, I faced this new challenger head on. I soon found that if I didn't overdo it with physical tasks every day, I wouldn't have as many episodes. If I did too much, it would trigger a seizure.

Therefore, I rested as much as I could with three children and got creative with my rambunctious, busy little people. Being practically on bedrest was no easy task, but I was determined to do what was best for my unborn baby. Good thing we had lots of cartoons available because we watched a lot of them. Since that wasn't something we usually did all the time, it was a treat for the girls. The only challenge was Callen, who was little enough that he wasn't interested in TV and needed lots of snuggles.

That winter, we were very relieved when I delivered a healthy little blond boy who we named Carter. He was so cute and even though he wasn't very big, he had chunky little legs. It was incredible to hold another perfect miracle from God in my arms. It was another crazy period of adjustment for all of us once we brought Carter home, since Callen and Carter were only fifteen months apart. But I couldn't have been happier. Despite the physical challenges I went through during my pregnancy, Jeff and I were so blessed to have four beautiful children. Each one looked so different, but my love for them was the same. I was fulfilling my dreams of having a large family with my wonderful husband.

Even though it was a lot of work, I felt like I was doing a good job taking care of everyone. Sure, it was overwhelming at times, but I loved every minute of it. There were days where I wasn't as patient as I would like, but I tried to enjoy the baby and toddler stages. Everyone loved to remind me that this stage would be over way too soon. With how hectic things could be, I didn't have much time to sit around and think about the seizures that I had thankfully left behind. I was too busy.

About one month after Carter was born, Jeff and I sat down to have an important discussion. Even though we had wanted a big family, Jeff and I both worried that my body couldn't handle another pregnancy. The seizures were very concerning and even though we were lucky to have four healthy babies, we were worried our luck would not continue. Also, I couldn't ignore my grumpiness that we blamed on pregnancy and post-pregnancy hormones. I just didn't feel like myself.

It seemed like I had either been pregnant or had a newborn for so long that we had just accepted this new "me" as normal. Perhaps, we thought, if my body could actually have the time to fully heal after having four kids so close together, then I would be able to recover and be back to my "old self" in no time.

Jeff and I prayed long and hard. As difficult as it was, we somehow knew that having more children would not be good for my body. I might not make it. We had been fortunate so far, but another baby might not make it, either.

Together, we took permanent measures for birth control. Quietly, I grieved for the children I would never bear.

CHAPTER 9

NOT GONNA FILL THOSE PRESCRIPTIONS

"I love you," I said as I kissed Jeff and gave him a quick hug before he left for work. It was barely 8am, but I'd already been up for a couple hours with four little ones. I winced in pain as another migraine came to the surface. I quickly got some medicine for myself, hoping I caught the migraine in time and the medicine would work. If I didn't, it would be another long day with a very bad headache.

With breakfast taken care of, I made my way up to the loft that was the children's playroom. This was where we spent most of our precious time together, playing and reading and dancing to our hearts' content. Despite the exhaustion of every moment of motherhood so far, I was incredibly grateful that I was able to be home with my kids every day. Things certainly weren't perfect and I spent most of the time covered in dried baby food, dirty laundry and occasional open-mouthed cat naps in front of Disney movies, but . . . life was good. (And eventually bedtime rolled around so I could finally breathe.)

But that morning, as I put away the last of the clean, dry dishes from breakfast, I noticed that my stomach was upset. I put a hand across my abdomen, wondering why I felt like I was going to be sick. Then a crash and several cries echoed from upstairs and I shook off the feeling. It'd happened yesterday morning, too, yes, but I had other stuff to worry about!

Lunchtime came and I fed all the kids, but didn't have much of an appetite for myself. I ate a banana so I would have something in my stomach, but it was hard to swallow. I gagged a little and ended up feeding the rest of the banana to Callen. More and more, I was having stomach discomfort and was having a hard time eating. Then, when nighttime came, I had a hard time falling asleep because I was having a weird internal itching sensation throughout my entire body. I snuggled up to Jeff in our bed, exhausted from the day.

"I am so itchy again! It's so weird. It feels like little bugs are crawling around under my skin. It's hard to explain," I vented to Jeff.

"Did you take some Benadryl?" Jeff asked.

"I tried that for two days and it didn't make the itching go away at all. I thought maybe I was having an allergy, but I don't think that's it. I'm also exhausted." I hated complaining to Jeff after he'd been gone working all day, but it felt good to talk through how I was feeling.

"Well, you do have four cute kids that you are running after. They keep you busy." Jeff laughed.

"True," I laughed with him, "but I think it's more than that. And lately, I haven't had an appetite. Once I actually eat, I'm super nauseated. And the kids have actually been sleeping through the night . . . all of them, which is a miracle. But I'm still so tired."

"You need to see the doctor," Jeff insisted. "I know how tough you are, honey, but I'm worried about you."

I gave him a worried smile. Even though our room was dark, I could still see the frustration in the lines on his forehead in the pale light of the moon shining through our window. He was probably right, even though I didn't want to admit it. *Just push through the pain,* I thought stubbornly. *That's what I've always done.*

"Please?" Jeff insisted and I sighed in defeat.

The next morning I asked Jeff if he had a family physician that he liked so I could make an appointment. I had been relatively healthy and hadn't needed to have a regular doctor since I had moved to Utah. Of course my kids had their pediatrician that I took them to and I had plenty of visits to my OB in the past few years. After the recommendation from Jeff, I made an appointment with my new primary care physician, then commenced the monumental task of finding child care for all my kids so I could go out to the small office building not far from our home. Once I sat down in the cool, quiet exam room, adjusting my seat on the paper-lined table, I was alone with my thoughts. Countless questions arose as to what these new, odd symptoms could mean.

The "episodes" or seizures are gone now that I'm not having any more children. But these other things just aren't normal. This has to be something else besides being exhausted all the time and not having time to exercise or do things for myself.

When the doctor came in, I began to explain what was going on: "I'm having this weird internal itching, migraines and bad headaches every day. There's also stomach aches, fatigue and I don't feel like myself anymore. I'm usually a pretty happy person, but I've been a little grumpy lately."

"Okay," he started. "Do you have any kids?" he asked, as he was taking notes.

I smiled widely. "Yes, I have four," I bragged, being the proud mama I was.

"How old are they?"

"Five and a half, four, two and a half and eighteen months. They are all pretty close." I was thrilled to have all these sweet children.

"Do you work, stay at home, or what does a regular day look like for you?" he questioned, as I wondered what he was getting at with all of these questions.

"Well, I am a stay-at-home mom, but I also do freelance graphic design from home while the kids are napping or sleeping at night. I have an old farmhouse that we have been fixing up for the last few years, so I do projects now and then."

The doctor's shoulders relaxed and he crossed his legs while he put my chart down. He calmly stated, "I think I know what's going on."

I sat up straight, a bright light of hope lit within me. *Wow, after telling him my symptoms and what I do from day to day, he knows what's going on? That's great. I'm going to be feeling better in no time!*

I leaned forward in anticipation to hear what he had discovered in such a short time.

"You have four small children, you work and seem to have a lot on your plate." He adjusted himself on the small stool, looking me right in the eye. "I think you are dealing with depression."

What? My eyebrows narrowed, my nose scrunched up and confusion filled my chest. *Depressed? This guy doesn't know me at all! I love having four small children and working. I'm not depressed.*

But instead of speaking up, I sat there silently as the doctor handed me two prescriptions. One was an antidepressant and the other was a sleeping medication, which was funny because I wasn't having any trouble sleeping.

As I got back in my car, I couldn't help feeling frustrated. After all, I didn't feel stressed out with what was on my plate. I wasn't feeling the best, but I wasn't feeling terrible either. I had always thrived being busy and I always wanted to work on the side while being a stay at home mom.

So, not satisfied or happy with my diagnosis, I decided to ignore the doctor and drove straight home instead of to the pharmacy. There was no way I was going to fill either of the prescriptions. A medicinal band aid wasn't what I was looking for; I wanted some real answers.

I continued to work and take care of my kids, taking them to the park and spending all my time with them. One day, as I was pushing them on the swings, I questioned my mental stability. I smiled at myself as I concluded that I wasn't depressed. I was happy with my life. I was living the life I had always dreamed of and I certainly knew I wasn't sad about it.

After keeping up my usual routine for a couple of weeks, I made another appointment with the same doctor. This time around, I was ready to stand up for myself. "I'm not depressed," I insisted. "But I know something else is going on. Can't you help me?" I glared at him, letting him know I wasn't going home until he helped me.

The doctor met my gaze and I was pretty sure he didn't know what to do with me. "Okay, Mrs. Peterson," he conceded. "Let's run some tests."

We started with blood work and had my gallbladder checked. That was when it was discovered that it was only functioning at 35%. My doctor informed me that even though the gallbladder doesn't heal itself, they wouldn't take it out until it was only functioning at 30%. That confused me, but I was glad that, as I waited for the right time to remove it, they had at least found something wrong. *Maybe that's why I'm not feeling well.*

Every other part of my body was also checked and the doctor told me that, other than my gallbladder, there was nothing wrong. On paper I was healthy, so I began to come to a conclusion that I didn't like at all: perhaps it really was just depression. It couldn't all be in my head . . . could it?

Without any other answers, I continued to push forward. My gallbladder was slowly getting worse, but life went back to "normal." I did my best to find time to work out and made healthy meals for my whole family. All the while, through every early morning with the kids and every play date with their friends, I ignored the fact that I still didn't feel good. Besides Jeff and some close family members, the world thought I was fine. I was developing some seriously good skills at faking it.

After about six months, I started to believe the idea that there wasn't anything wrong with me. I was pretty good at pretending I was happy, even though that wasn't always the truth. Instead, I kept praying and tried to listen to where God was guiding me. Every time, I was told to go back to my doctor.

So, I went back and suffered through a new slew of tests. Finally, this time around he diagnosed me with fibromyalgia, then referred me to a gastroenterologist for my stomach problems. Grateful for some new answers that might finally bring me peace, I embraced the idea that these doctors would help solve my problems. Faith continued to guide me.

CHAPTER 10

I LOVE BREAD

My gastroenterologist turned out to be one of the nicest doctors I knew. Something about his calm demeanor and willingness to listen made me break down in his office during our first appointment. With great patience, he watched me cry like crazy as I shared all of my symptoms for what felt like the millionth time.

"You know what, Brita?" he began, a knowing look in his eye. "We're going to test you for celiac disease."

I'd never heard of this before, but by then I was open to any and all options. As they prepared for the test, the doctor also decided to order an endoscopy and colonoscopy, just to be thorough. Jeff and the kids had to wait around for a while afterward since I took my sweet time coming out of anesthesia. I must have needed a good nap! A few days later when I got a phone call from the gastroenterologist's office, I expected them to say that everything was fine. Instead, the nurse said that my test results in fact showed that I had celiac disease.

Shocked, I stepped back from the play room where the kids were having a blast together, not expecting to need a quiet place to hear such news. As I held tight to the phone, listening to the nurse explain what my next steps were, I felt uneasiness creep over me. I'd never had an actual *disease* before. And even more so, this was something I knew absolutely nothing about.

I cleared my throat and took a shaky breath. "Yes," I answered the nurse. "Let's set up a follow-up appointment with the specialist." After I'd managed that, I hung up and began to cry.

Luckily, my family was in town during that beautiful summer week, so I had all the support in the world. And, after talking more with my doctor, I learned that if I cut out gluten (wheat, barley and rye) from my diet, my body would likely heal itself and I would be fine. *Well, I can do that,* I thought. *But . . . how can I survive without bread? I really, really love bread!*

Shortly after my diagnosis, celiac disease became very popular. There were so many gluten-free options that became available to the public, sometimes to help those with the disease and other times just for those who wanted to change their diet of their own choice. It seemed like celiac disease was known by practically everyone and most people seemed to know someone who had it. Thankfully, it seemed I had been diagnosed at a time when more and more tasty, gluten-free options were being created.

I began the overwhelming process of reworking every single thing I ate (which included taking out a lot of items that I loved). Gluten-free options were pretty expensive, so I decided that I would just get them for me and continue to feed my family the food they were used to. After about a month, I started to feel a little better, but none of my debilitating symptoms were fully going away. My doctor shared with me that it could take a whole year of my new diet before I'd be back to my old self.

The next step in my journey was to see an allergist who could determine if there were any particular foods I was allergic to. Luckily, my allergen test did not show that I had any food allergies. So instead, I began an elimination diet, only eating a limited number of foods and then adding new ones to see if anything bothered me. I decided to start by cutting out dairy because I read that a lot of people with celiac disease might be lactose intolerant. That seemed to help a little, but it was really just another form of torture. If there was anything I loved more than bread, it was cheese, ice cream and pretty much any dairy items. But at least I could eat fruit, vegetables, rice, meat, candy and a bunch of things that made me happy. I could still function.

One day, the kids and I sat down to play a game of cards. It was close to bedtime and we sometimes settled down together by enjoying a relaxing game before I got them all off to their rooms. Jeff was working late, but I knew he'd be home soon. We gathered around the table, but as soon as the cards were handed out, I knew something was wrong.

The kids were laughing, excited to play UNO. Their laughter irritated me, which didn't make sense; I usually loved hearing their cute laughs. Landan put a blue two on a green card and it made me uncharacteristically annoyed. I tried controlling my voice as I moved her card. "Remember, you have to put the same color or number on the cards in the pile."

Landan gave me a smile and a giggle as she replaced the blue card with one of her green ones. Taylor was next and she put a red card on the green one. Anger was brewing and my fuse was getting short. The kids were being silly and it was making me so agitated. I was aware that this wasn't normal, but for some reason I couldn't control my feelings. The kids went a few more rounds, having a good time, but each time they made a mistake, my words got more and more grumpy. The looks on their faces were so sad and they were even more disappointed when I stopped the game before it was over.

"Alright, kids, it's time for bed. Go brush your teeth. Landan and Taylor, can you help the boys brush theirs, please?"

"But our game isn't over!" they all cried out.

"Yes it is!" I snapped. "Everyone brush your teeth and it's time for bed." The words came out sharper than I wanted and it was everything I could do to not hit the kids. Why was this happening? I was doing the best I could to control these feelings that were growing more intense inside of me and I hoped I wouldn't lose my temper completely.

With shaky hands, I flipped off the last light switch and shut the last bedroom door. I stumbled downstairs to the quiet family room, in utter shock and terror. Gathering one of the sofa pillows against my chest, I fell apart. Tears poured onto the cushion as I thought, *I'm so grateful I didn't hurt any of the kids! But why do I feel so out of control? I've been doing such a good job with my new diet . . . is it possible I ate something I shouldn't have? Could food make me feel like this?*

When Jeff got home, all my feelings rose to the surface again. He set down his bag on the kitchen counter and tried to come over to hug me, no doubt because of the tear stains on my face. But I backed away from him, shaking my head. "I don't know what is wrong with me!" I cried. "For some reason, tonight I've been furious! I could have thrown each of the kids against the wall and they didn't even do anything wrong."

"Brita," he began, holding out his arms trying to hold me, "it's okay."

"Don't come close," I insisted, stepping even further back. "I just want to hit you."

I shoved his arm away that he was trying to wrap around me. "I'm being serious. Don't touch me. I don't want to hurt you."

Alarm spread across Jeff's face and I could tell he was realizing something really was wrong. That kind of behavior was *so* not me. I was always very affectionate and loved getting hugged by my husband.

I cleared my throat and shut my eyes for a moment. "The kids are in bed," I said quietly, "but I'd love for you to check on them. I need to be by myself for a bit."

I walked outside alone, through the grass and settled on our cement pad under the basketball hoop, leaning against the pole. I gazed out across our field through blurry eyes, to see the magnificent mountains in the distance, though this time they didn't cheer me up. I loved this spot because no one could see me; I could hide out away from the world. I cried for as long as the hot tears would come. Finally, when most of my anger and confusion had spilled out, I called my mom and filled her in on what I was experiencing. She listened and comforted me. The tears dried upon my face and my mood lifted. Eventually, I went back inside, thankful for the comfort of Jeff's open arms waiting for me.

A few days later, I found out that I had indeed accidentally eaten some item with gluten in the house. It turned out that if I did have something that I didn't have a tolerance for, it would put me in a nasty, sick state for four to seven days. My kids started teasing me, saying their mom "would turn into The Hulk if she wasn't careful." After about a week passed, I'd be left with fatigue and stomach pain.

What a nightmare.

Finally, I couldn't take it anymore. I decided that all gluten needed to be removed from the house. It hurt my heart to clean out our pantry of all the yummy things my family loved to eat, but Jeff was so supportive, as always. We embarked on the adventure of figuring out how to bake treats that I could eat and everyone else would hopefully enjoy as much as what they'd been so used to.

Unfortunately, a lot of the gluten-free baking recipes I came across tasted like styrofoam and finding a decent blend of ingredients took forever. I had very patient taste-testers in my children and eventually I found a blend of tapioca starch and white rice flour that worked pretty well. Once I had that base to go off of, I created some delicious recipes, including my German Chocolate Cake. That one was gluten, dairy and soy free! I wasn't much of a baker to begin with, so I always swelled with pride when my little ones gobbled up the goodies that I could also sit and enjoy with them. Going gluten free wasn't so bad after all.

That fall when the kids were in school again, I noticed that Landan would come home with headaches and stomachaches. It was so bad that I took her to the doctor, crying in pain, but they couldn't find anything wrong with my six-year-old girl. Then Taylor had stomach issues, too, as well as Callen and Carter (once he was old enough to eat solid food). When we had them tested, none of the kids had celiac disease, for which I was thankful.

That's when I decided to talk with the school and with my kids' friends' families, to share with them that we were 100% gluten-free at home. They needed to have the same diet at school and while visiting their friends so they wouldn't get sick. Eventually, when the new diet was stuck to, Jeff and I realized everyone was physically feeling much better. Our house was free of headaches and tummy aches!

After six long months, I began to feel really comfortable with the gluten-free diet. I was so hopeful that my body would heal and I would get back to being my old self. Even though I had a lot of good moments during those months, much to my dismay, I did not start feeling completely better. That led me back to the doctor and then to different specialists to find out if there was something else wrong with me. Were they missing something?

Honestly, every doctor I saw acted like I was crazy. I would tell them how tired I was, the internal itching I still felt and my other weird symptoms, but they acted like I just liked the attention of going to the doctor. Little did they know, I hated going to the doctor, but I hated it more that I felt awful all the time. Without the energy to do anything, I found myself wondering if there was anyone else in the world who was going through the same frustrations as me.

I wished I could talk to someone who understood me. I did go to a celiac support group and it was great, but I still didn't feel like I could relate to anyone. It seemed like most people there had the "regular" symptoms and it was discouraging for me.

Because my doctor admitted that he didn't know what else to do for me in the spring of 2010, he referred me to more doctors where I received some bad news. I'd been having some new symptoms that included being thirsty all the time and peeing all the time. After ruling out diabetes, this time he referred me to a urologist.

When I told the urologist all my symptoms and told him I had celiac disease, he immediately said, "We treat a lot of women with celiac disease who also have this condition."

What condition? I thought nervously. *Do I have something else?*

I was diagnosed with interstitial cystitis, a bladder condition also known as IC/PBS (painful bladder syndrome). This condition was sometimes helped with yet another diet change, so I found out that eliminating acidic foods was what I needed to do next. I was given a list of foods that I could and could not eat. On top of cutting out gluten, dairy and soy, I now had to cut out fruit, chocolate and a bunch of other things. The list of what my body could tolerate was getting even smaller. Push through the pain was what I always told myself and I tried to stay positive now. Cutting out food seemed like a relatively small sacrifice to potentially feel better.

Shortly after that diagnosis, I had my uterus scoped because I was having some girl problems, some of which included heavy bleeding. The OB found extremely huge varicose veins from my ovaries to my uterus. There wasn't much they could do, but they suggested I get a hysterectomy, which I didn't want. Even though I was done having kids, I didn't want to be on hormones the rest of my life.

While the doctor was doing the scope of my uterus, they found that my appendix was shriveled, white and hard, which was very unusual. The OB had another surgeon come in for a second opinion and they both agreed that they should take my appendix out right then. I woke up without an appendix and the unhappy decision to make about needing a hysterectomy.

It was more apparent now than ever before why I didn't like going to the doctor; every time I went in for answers, I always ended up with more problems. I felt like my health was just getting worse and worse. Then I asked myself a question that scared me more than anything: would I ever be healthy again?

After recovering from having my appendix removed, I went to get a second opinion about getting a hysterectomy. That wasn't something I was ready to jump into if I didn't really need it. This doctor first put me on progesterone to see if that would help and instead of the hysterectomy, he recommended a procedure called an ablation, which would burn the walls of my uterus, to potentially stop my bleeding.

That seemed like a better option than a hysterectomy, so after Jeff and I discussed it, we decided it was worth a try. It was one of the most painful things I had ever done. They told me I would most likely be up and back to normal activities within one day, but, of course, I was in severe pain and vomited for three days before I started feeling better. When I was up and out of bed, I was happy to discover it had worked! The bleeding had stopped completely.

Maybe it's okay to have real hope this time. From now on, things will just get better.

CHAPTER 11

MUSIC VIDEOS AND NEW YORK

Music and exercise were incredibly important parts of my life. With my current limitations, however, it was hard for me to stay active. I pushed myself, as usual, to do as many workouts as I could. When I started having issues with my feet, I went to see a local podiatrist. We started chatting about my passion for music and the songs I'd written whenever I had time.

"You know," he began during one of our appointments, "I have a patient who was part of a popular singing group in the '50s and '60s. I'm pretty sure he produces albums for new artists nowadays. I should introduce you to Bob."

Although I was nervous, it was exciting to set up a meeting with Bob. I'd never thought about talking with a professional in the music industry about what I wrote and played and sung just for myself. But once I met Bob, he made me feel at ease as I sat down and performed one of my originals for him at his brother's big, beautiful home. Bob, who was getting along in years, sat his thin body in a chair next to the piano and listened intently.

"Intriguing," he murmured when I finished, nodding his head. "But I want you to work on this part . . ." He gave me an assignment of how to rewrite a section of the song and to come back the following week. That wasn't something I was used to doing, but I was serious about where this could take my music so I found myself back at his door by the deadline he'd given.

For the next few months, I met every instructional challenge that Bob sent my way. Finally, he was happy with the results and agreed to produce my CD . . . for free!

For the next year and a half, I faced the task of recording my demo at the studio downtown. My energy levels were so low that this was a lot harder than it should have been. Many days I could barely get into the sound booth, let alone muster the strength to sing. *This is my dream,* I told myself with determination every time I wanted to quit. *I've always wanted to do this, so I'm going to see it through.*

Most nights, I would put my kids in bed, kiss my husband goodbye and head to the studio for a late-night recording session. For a person who was still trying to heal my body from celiac disease and all the unknown, unsolvable problems I was also facing, this was a rough schedule. I refused to back down, some days crying alone while driving to and from the studio, but eventually I was able to get my demo done.

It was such an amazing accomplishment and my family celebrated with me as I unbelievably held the CD in my hands for the first time. Bob was so encouraging and believed in me every step of the way. With Bob's help, I started sending out the demos to record companies. I don't know if it was the fact that I'd just achieved one of my life goals at the age of thirty, but I was actually feeling pretty good. Jeff even commented one day that I was starting to act like myself again. I couldn't help but agree and dared to let myself have a bit of hope. *Maybe I'm on the road to recovery this time! It would be so wonderful to finally be healthy again.*

Bob made plans for me to start performing and we were getting my show ready, which consisted of live shows performing with the local talent that Bob was friends with. I was impressed with all the local celebrities he knew personally and that he wanted me to be a part of that scene. It was overwhelming and exciting. We even put together a music video in a couple of weeks with some incredible friends of mine. The demo was called "Bree—100% Original." Bob encouraged me to name the album *Bree* since my name was hard to pronounce, so I went with that. I couldn't have been prouder to have it finished.

In the meantime, Jeff had been working hard at his sales job. One evening that summer when the sun was burning bright colors into the horizon, Jeff came home from work with a big announcement: with a wide grin, he shared that he'd hit one of his biggest sales goals for the quarter. His reward was a bonus trip to New York City!

As I set down the dishes I was drying next to the sink, I ran over and gave him an enormous hug. "I am so proud of you, babe!" I gushed, planting a kiss on his cheek.

"Do you want to come with me?" he asked with a wink.

Excitement rushed through me as I pulled back and met his eyes. New York City was always somewhere I wanted to go. I practically jumped over to the phone to call my parents and see if they would watch the kids. They were always so supportive and were more than willing to babysit. It was so fun to plan our trip, but I couldn't help feeling a bit nervous.

How will I feel when we get there? I've got to get on a plane, go to a big city and try entirely new things. I had been doing okay lately with my health, but my energy levels and anxiety could be an issue at any time. *Please,* I prayed every night leading up to our departure, *please let Jeff and I enjoy our precious time together in the city.*

The relief I felt on the plane was unexpected. I was surprised by how light I felt knowing that for the next few days I didn't have to take care of anyone but myself on this trip. As fiercely as I loved my sweet babies, I didn't have the energy to keep up with them all the time. Jeff and I could rest if needed, go see sights, or do whatever we wanted and we didn't have anyone else to dictate our plans. I realized then that this was a much-needed break for me. Maybe I would return rejuvenated.

I was worried at first that I wouldn't be able to find any gluten-free restaurants, but my phone didn't disappoint, as it led us to some fabulous restaurants and bakeries. Food was not an issue for us. We found one particular burger joint that we visited several times. During each of our adventures, I couldn't help watching my husband. Jeff was so cute as he excitedly explored the city with me. It made my heart soar to see him enjoying himself alongside me. It seemed that his burdens were also lightened on this trip.

Every time we sat down for a meal or to catch our breath, I made a point to look into his eyes and really appreciate how amazing of a man he was. Jeff did so many things for our family at home. He worked, took care of our family financially, helped take care of the kids once he came home and was a huge support to me.

What a wonderful man I have sitting in front of me. How did I get so lucky?

I wished our carefree, fun time in the magic of New York City could have lasted forever, but soon we were back to real life, with kids to take care of. Still inspired by how well I'd handled our trip, I tried getting in shape again by going to a CrossFit class that Jeff had been going to. I didn't have a lot of energy, but I didn't know what else to do with my conundrum: the doctors kept acting like nothing was wrong with me and that I just needed to get into great shape.

When I arrived at the gym, I was fully prepared to not hold back. Even though it was hard, I still completed every rep and every interval in the hour-long class. At the end of the session, I was shaking so badly that I could hardly walk to the car. My face was bright red when I glanced in the rearview mirror. With trembling hands, I picked up my phone, realizing I was so weak I might not be able to drive home.

"Umm, Jeff," I began when he picked up, "I think I might die." I let out a weak chuckle.

Jeff and I had a good laugh and I sat in my car for a while as I caught my breath so I could drive home. I was able to finish two weeks of CrossFit work-out twice a week before my body couldn't keep up and I sadly had to stop. I was disappointed because I loved the challenge of the workouts.

I knew something was still *off* in my body. Every night, I prayed that one day I would find someone who could discover what it was. I began to think that two weeks of CrossFit wasn't the best idea when my body wouldn't do what it needed to do in order to get through every day with the kids. My energy was gone once again.

Frustration filled me again when, crazily, I could barely walk around the house. If I did the simplest chore, like trying to load the dishwasher, I got so winded that I could hardly function. Most days, my kids sat on my bed with me and watched a lot of movies. Jeff quickly saw how bad things were for me and grudgingly, I decided to go back to the doctor.

CHAPTER 12

TICKING TIME BOMB

"Y ou have Hashimoto's disease, Brita."

I blinked, giving the specialist before me a bewildered look. *Another disease?* I couldn't believe it. I was told that my thyroid was enlarged and I needed to see an endocrinologist for further testing. Determined to get more answers from a different doctor once more, I set up an appointment.

However, when I got to the endocrinologist's office, he hardly looked at me. Instead, I sat across from him in his spacious office, my medical file open on his ornate desk. He sighed, pushed a hand through his white hair and turned a page in front of him. Then he flung the page over his shoulder. I stared, confused, as the paper fluttered to the floor. Each time he read a page, he threw it onto the ground dismissively. I had never seen a doctor go through a file like this and was at a loss for words.

Eventually, when my entire medical history lay in a disorganized pile on the floor, he glanced at me over his dark glasses.

"You don't have a thyroid problem," he declared, arrogance in his tone.

What? "But," I objected, anger edging into my tone, "I was just told I have Hashimoto's disease. That's why I'm here!"

"Nope. Not a thyroid problem," he insisted and took a seat behind his desk. "Tell me everything that's going on."

I couldn't tell if he actually listened to me as I listed all of my weird symptoms for what felt like the millionth time.

"Has anyone ever checked your heart?"

"No," I snapped back, unable to hide my frustration anymore. "I've never had heart problems."

The doctor let out a huge sigh and said, "Well, I really don't think there is anything wrong with you." He stared at me over his glasses, annoyed, like I was wasting his precious time.

What a weird guy.

"Because of my expertise, I have to check everything out or I could get into trouble," he informed me. "It doesn't seem like anything is wrong with you, but I will send you to get some tests, so you know nothing is wrong. Looks like you have good insurance, so why not?"

Defeated, I went ahead and scheduled more tests. Afterward, I felt awful for an entire week. No matter what I did, I was grumpy, sad and exhausted.

At the end of the week I had a follow-up appointment with the endocrinologist.

"Well," the doctor announced, "it looks like you have Hashimoto's disease, an autoimmune disease where the body attacks the thyroid."

My jaw dropped slightly as I stared at the man who had told me a week ago that I *didn't* have a thyroid problem. Of course, he didn't apologize for telling me before that nothing was wrong with me. Instead, he gave me the information like he knew what was plaguing my body the entire time.

So, I was now on thyroid medication trying to find the right dose for my body. The only thing left looming in the near future was my heart test. At that point, every time I went to the doctor, it seemed I was getting diagnosed with something, so I was fearful this heart test would show another problem. *I really hope I'm wrong.*

The day before my heart test, a friend of mine called to check in on me. As we chatted, she said, "So, my sister-in-law has had similar symptoms. You need to make sure they do the bubble test during your echocardiogram."

"Okay . . . I have no idea what that is," I replied, "but thank you!"

The next morning when I showed up to the lab, I made sure to get the technician's attention. While he was getting me ready, he asked, "So, are we doing the bubble study today?"

I looked at him, surprised and glad it had come up. "Umm . . . yes, sure. Let's do the bubble thing."

An IV was placed in my arm so the technician could send air and a small amount of saline through my veins as he took pictures. Afterward, the technician shared, "Well, you do have a good amount of bubbles going in the wrong place. Looks like you may have what's called an atrial septal defect, or ASD."

"What does that mean?" I exclaimed in complete shock. I couldn't accept that I might have a heart problem.

"It just means that you have a hole in the wall that separates the top two chambers of your heart." He smiled at me like he was giving me some kind of good news.

"So, will I need heart surgery?" I demanded nervously. I came into the test that morning almost sure they wouldn't find anything and now I was worried about the function of my heart.

"You will have to talk to your doctor about the test results. I'm not allowed to tell you any more." He gave me a sympathetic glance.

Well, thanks a lot, I thought with exasperation. *That didn't help me at all. Now I'm just freaking out, wondering what is going on with my heart.*

My cardiologist had to do further testing to show how much blood was flowing in the wrong wall of my heart. In the meantime, I couldn't get over the fact that I might have a heart problem. I was young and an athlete, so it didn't make sense. Things got worse when I found out that my next test results were pretty bad and that I'd likely need surgery to correct the problem.

Expecting to schedule surgery with my cardiologist, I was shocked when he looked over my chart once more and just sent me home with aspirin instead. "You're not a candidate for surgery, Brita," he told me shortly.

"I don't understand," I replied slowly.

"You need to have an episode of some sort, like a stroke, to prove that there is an issue here," he explained. "And you won't get approved for surgery if we also don't have a neurologist prove the benefits of a procedure."

I didn't know what to do next. The test results showed I had a problem with my heart, even the technicians seemed confident that I needed to get help, but to my doctor, apparently, nothing could be done right away. That's when I knew I needed a second opinion. Because I'd seen a neurologist during my weird pregnancy issues, I went back to Dr. Vincent, hopeful that she could help me.

Dr. Vincent looked at all of my test results that were sent to her and she asked, "When did you have your surgery?"

"I haven't had surgery," I replied, irritated. "The cardiologist I was going to said I didn't have a heart problem."

Panic blossomed in her brown eyes. She stared at me with concern for a few seconds, then reread my test results. "You definitely have a heart problem!"

As she flipped through all my paperwork, she continued, "I have a different cardiologist I want you to go see. His name is Dr. Ganellen. He is great and I have worked with him in the past. Get in as soon as you can. He and I will discuss the next steps for you."

Dr. Vincent then explained that this new information made her worry the "seizures" they thought I'd had during my last two pregnancies could have actually been mini strokes or TIAs.

My throat went dry when she got very serious and leaned closer to me. I didn't realize I was holding my breath until I let out a big sigh after she spoke, "You need to go home, put your feet up and try to get all of the stress out of your life. I hate to tell you this, but you are a ticking time bomb, Brita. I am worried you could have a major stroke before we can get you into surgery."

Normally, I would have burst into tears at such news, but I was so dumbfounded I couldn't process what she had just said. With four small children at home, there wasn't an easy way to be stress-free. So many thoughts raced through my head. *A ticking time bomb? Did she think telling me something like that was going to make me feel better?* Now I was really freaking out and couldn't wait to get to my car so I could let the tears fall. Immediately, I called Jeff and tried to tell him the news as I cried.

With the help of many wonderful people around me, I was able to rest as I waited for my insurance to approve the surgery that Dr. Ganellen and Dr. Vincent wanted to perform. People from my church and my Aunt Regina came and cleaned, made meals, watched the kids and helped us in so many ways. Aunt Regina showed up time and time again and I will be forever thankful for all the help she gave me and my family during such a challenging time. My good friends, Sandi and Renee, came to surprise me with a beautiful yellow and blue quilt that they made me as a reminder of their friendship and love.

They were incredible friends, constantly buoying me up, helping me through the hard days. With what little energy I had, I hugged them fiercely and was so thankful. Lately, I hadn't been able to be the friend I wanted to be for them, but that didn't stop them from showing me that they were there for me no matter what.

I felt helpless and prayed constantly that I could get through surgery and be able to live and take care of my greatest blessings, my children. I wasn't afraid to die, but the thought of leaving my children without a mother was my greatest fear.

Finally, more details came in: my procedure was scheduled for March, two months away and it couldn't come soon enough. Luckily, I didn't need open heart surgery, but I was still terribly nervous. The procedure was going to be done by a catheter going through a large vein in my leg, where they would place an umbrella-like device to open and plug the hole once it was in the correct spot.

My parents drove from Oregon to be with us. Jeff and my dad came to the hospital with me while my mom stayed home to take care of the kids. Even though it really freaked me out, I was awake and watched my whole heart procedure on a computer screen. Even though it upset my weak stomach and I didn't really want to be awake, the medication they gave me helped a lot. The drugs took away most of my memories of that day, for which I was thankful.

Afterward, I was told that the surgery went well. I had to lie on my back for a whole hour without moving. Still being a little loopy when the nurse came in, I had to confess, "Umm, I really need to go to the bathroom."

The nurse escorted my husband and Dad out of the room. When she was back at my bedside, she said, "Well, here's the deal since you can't get up: we can either put in a catheter, or I can put a pink bucket under you and you can go." She smiled as she mentioned option number two.

That was an easy choice for me. "I do not want a catheter if I can help it. Can we try the bucket?"

Carefully, the nurse helped me raise my hips as she slid the bucket under me. *Talk about stage fright!* It felt so weird to be letting go of my urine while lying on my back, but I was in so much pain. Instantly, I felt relief as I began to empty my bladder in the bucket.

"Oh, dear," the nurse gasped. The bucket's almost full. Are you almost done?"

Neither of us were prepared for how full my bladder was. I never would have thought one bladder could fill a pink hospital bucket.

We both started laughing hysterically as the bucket overflowed. I couldn't move and I suddenly found myself swimming in my own pee. Finally, I was done and the nurse sloshed the overflowing bucket out of the way. I was so wet and couldn't help but feel disgusted with the situation. My nurse was awesome and cleaned everything up while I felt like a helpless little child.

She was so kind and after such a stressful surgery, it felt good to laugh even if it was terribly embarrassing and really gross. Gratitude filled me that I had such an incredible nurse with a great sense of humor. I hoped that I was one of her "oh my gosh, guess what happened at work today" stories that she told her family that night.

Once Jeff and my dad were back in the room, they were both trying to cheer me up. Dad told one of his funny jokes, trying to lighten the mood for all of us. Even though I wasn't in the joking mood, I could see the worry in his eyes and I appreciated the way he always tried to make me feel better.

Not long after I was in the recovery room, Dr. Ganellen came to check on me. He briefed us on the successful surgery. "Usually when I repair these types of holes, it only takes about thirty seconds for me to find the hole. But you were a lot different, Brita. It took me a good two minutes to find your hole, which was really abnormal. It was in a very unusual, hard to find place."

I glanced over at Jeff, concerned as the doctor continued.

"But, finally, I did find it and closed it up with a device like an umbrella. The surgery took a little longer because the first device we put in was too small. We had to take it out and get a bigger size. When I finally found the hole, it was twice the size we thought it was at about fourteen millimeters, which is pretty big."

I was still a little groggy from the drugs, but I was so thankful that I had an amazing surgeon who took his time and made sure to fix my heart.

"You are very lucky that you haven't had any major problems from such a large ASD," Dr. Ganellen added. "I can't believe that you got through childbirth four times, because bearing down is the worst thing you could have done for your heart condition."

I chuckled a little and teased, "So, the two weeks of CrossFit I did a few months ago before I found out about my heart problem probably wasn't a good idea?"

Dr. Ganellen shook his head and gave a sad smile as he responded, "No, that was not a good idea. You are lucky you are still alive."

I was pretty sure he didn't think I was funny. But I was happy that, for once, I had gotten some answers to a problem *and* a solution, too. Now I knew why I felt so terrible after each CrossFit workout and I was hoping this was the answer to why my body wasn't functioning well for the last few years.

He reassured me that recovery was pretty easy and I would be feeling back to myself in a week. It was such a relief to know that what was probably causing so many of my problems was now fixed. I was confident that this was why I had been feeling so bad. I couldn't wait to get through the next week and then start feeling amazing again.

When I got home, however, things were more difficult than anticipated. I was very sore and exhausted. I couldn't even get out of bed. Plus, I found that horrible migraines were triggered.

The second day after surgery, I was sitting in bed when all of a sudden my right arm started going numb and the right side of my face felt weird. I awkwardly texted my mom to come into my room, since she was still staying at our house taking care of me and my kids while Jeff went back to work.

By the time she came in to see me, the right side of my face was numb, I couldn't speak very well and my right leg was slowly getting numb. My mom called the cardiologist's office and they told her to take me to the ER immediately.

Thankfully, my wonderful neighbor came to watch my kids while my mom took me to the hospital. Jeff met us there and with my husband at my side giving me strength, we waited for news from the ER doctor.

CHAPTER 13

A STRANGER MOVES IN

Relief washed over me as the latest news we received wasn't as bad as I thought: the ER doctor shared that I wasn't having a stroke. *Thank goodness!* It was just a really horrible migraine with similar symptoms to stroke. I sighed with relief; migraines I could manage and had been tackling for a long time. And my body was still figuring out how to function with a healthy heart.

I'm a fighter, I told myself as we headed home. Fresh determination solidified my resolve. *I can do this.* I gathered all the kids into a hug the minute I got in the door, ready to once again conquer the pain and do my best to get back to exercising. Without that hole in my heart, I wanted to play at the park with my family and do as much as I could with each passing day.

Four days later, I opened my eyes before my alarm went off, which was a rare occurrence nowadays. I glanced around my dark room, then over at Jeff, who was still passed out. I treasured these quiet moments I had before the house was all awake. I closed my eyes again, not to sleep, but to say a silent prayer of gratitude.

Dear Father, thank You for my health. Thank You for the renewed energy I am receiving. Thank You so much for guiding me to the right doctors who have helped me so much. I am so grateful that I am still here, living and breathing. I am so thankful to be a mother of these wonderful children. Thank You . . .

Before I could say any more, my alarm went off and it was time to get the kids up and ready for school. I dismissed the alarm and slowly climbed the stairs to wake each sweet child. Smiles greeted me as they all got ready for school and met me in the kitchen for cereal.

My mom seemed surprised to see me up, since she had been helping out with the morning routine for a couple weeks. I gave her a warm smile to let her know I was good and she grinned back. Jeff came in shortly after, kissing my cheek and asking, "How are you today?"

"I actually feel good and I don't have a headache. It's really nice!"

I saw the relief wash over Jeff's face as he went to get ready for work. After hugs and kisses, my mom and I dropped the kids off at school and decided to stop by a nearby park for a short walk. Even though I was pretty slow while my mom and I chatted, it felt wonderful to be out in nature moving my body.

"It's great walking out here after a rough couple weeks," I stated, even though I was already winded from our short walk. I glanced around at the park, noticing the flowers in bloom and the green grass that beckoned me to come lie on it. My ears focused on the chirping birds overhead and I smiled at their sweet songs dancing above my head. I felt a new excitement for life and all the simple things around me.

"Yes, it's good to see you out of bed and feeling a little better. You had me worried," Mom replied.

Suddenly, my feet stopped in the middle of the path. It hadn't dawned on me until that moment how scared my mom must have been with everything I'd been facing lately. I know if one of my children was going through this, I would have been incredibly stressed out, to say the least.

Up until that moment, I hadn't thought about her perspective at all; I was so worried about my kids and my health, I hadn't given much thought to Mom's feelings. My love for my mom had grown even more when I took the time to realize her key role in my life. The dedication and love she always showered on me and my family was so comforting.

"Thanks so much for being here, Mom," I said, catching her full attention. "I really appreciate all you have done for us. It was so nice not having to worry about the kids while I was in surgery. You are always so great with them." I looked her straight in the eyes, so grateful to have such a supportive mother and family.

Mom's eyes were teary as she leaned in to give me a hug while responding back. "I'm just so glad you are okay." I knew she was trying to be tough and not cry. She swallowed hard and didn't say any more, but she didn't have to. I could feel her tenderness and love that she always shared with me.

Slowly, I was able to do more and more. I was sad to say goodbye to my mother, but I will be forever thankful that both she and my dad were able to make the time to be with us in that awful time. They helped us so much and it was such an important part of my healing to have them take care of our family.

My body was finally getting used to the new device that was in my heart. It was a slow process but, week by week, I felt small improvements. It was an amazing feeling. I had, most likely, been born with this heart condition and my body had never functioned the right way, even though I was a dedicated athlete. I imagined myself an even better athlete, had the doctors found this problem when I was young. The strain of my pregnancies exacerbated the weakness in my heart and I was lucky to be alive. I felt that heart surgery, celiac disease and Hashimoto's were the reasons for all my health problems and now I would finally start feeling better. It was a great feeling!

What a blessing! I knew God was watching out for me. I felt so guided to each new doctor that found and fixed my problems. I was very humbled through this experience as I knew that my life truly was in God's hands. Through much prayer, I was guided to the right doctors and I was healing. It was such a gift.

Not long after I was healing and beginning to feel stronger, it was brought to Jeff's and my attention that there was a twenty-one-year-old girl in our church who needed drastic help. The girl's mother had passed away in January and she didn't have anywhere to go. Many church members were doing as much for her as they could, but she was pregnant and alone and needed a safe place to stay.

When my husband and I heard about this girl's story, we began praying to know if and how we could help her. After much prayer, we felt like she could move in with us even though I was still recovering from my heart surgery. We had to do a little remodeling and rearranging to make space for her. Jeff and I prepared our children for a stranger to come live with us. We didn't know this girl and she didn't know us, but we were anxious to meet her.

I took a deep breath and reminded myself that this kind of thing was something that came natural for us. Both Jeff and I had grown up in service-oriented families, so we were always helping and serving people however we could. That included giving individuals a place to stay if needed, opening our hearts and homes to whoever deserved a little extra love. It was like second nature for us to have this strong desire to help.

When Nicole arrived at our door, with my friend Cindy, all I could see was long brown hair. Her head was bent toward the ground and I could feel the sadness coming from her as I watched her slow, small steps enter our house. Her eyes never looked up at me even when I said, "Hi Nicole, I'm Brita, it's nice to meet you."

Nicole glanced up shyly and nervously smiled without saying a word. Jeff, who is normally very social, could see that Nicole needed space and he said a soft hi as I showed Nicole to her room.

Nicole moved in with us in April 2012 and she was very much to herself. She would hardly come out of her room at all. The pregnancy made her quite ill so it wasn't easy for her to get out of bed. She was so heartbroken from her mother's death and was consumed in depression. She would mostly sleep all day and come out at night when we were in bed so she didn't have to interact with us.

It was very hard to see someone so sad, breaking our hearts to see her this way. Watching her, it made all of my trials seem so small. One night, I couldn't sleep and was in the kitchen getting a drink when Nicole came in to fill her craving. I started with small talk and told her how happy we were that she was living with us. She looked at me surprised and said, "Really, you like having me here?"

"Yes, I mean we don't even see you, so you are the best house mate." I smiled jokingly hoping she would warm up to me.

Nicole smiled and relaxed and we began talking and eventually, Nicole opened up to me about her hard past. She cried as she told me about losing her mom, not long after her sister passed away. She confided in me about her drug-addicted ex-boyfriend, the father of her baby and how she didn't want him to be a part of the baby's life.

She had held so much in for so long, I could feel the tension lift off of her as her shoulders softened and she relaxed into the chair for the first time since I had met her. I felt a deep connection to her as she shared her vulnerability with me and we became family in one night. I cried as she told me her story.

As she spoke, Nicole rubbed her growing belly. She was due in July and it was already the middle of May. There wasn't that much time left for her to prepare for the little girl she was carrying. She had been through so much abuse and pain and now she had to decide what to do with her baby.

It wasn't hard for my heart to understand exactly what she was feeling when she shared her deep pain with me. In fact, something inside me related to what she was saying, which was weird because I had never been through anything like her current circumstances. My empathetic nature grieved along with her and we created an unbreakable bond.

At that time, she was planning to keep her baby and I told her that she could stay with us as long as she wanted and that we were her family now. We would support her in any way that she needed. "Can I give you a hug?" I asked hesitantly since I knew how much she liked being alone.

"I would love that," Nicole replied and I pulled her in for a long hug where we both soaked each other's shoulders with tears.

Three weeks went by and Nicole and I had become such good friends. She was even coming out of her room during the day, getting to know the kids and Jeff. Because she hadn't had many positive male figures in her life, it took her longer to warm up to Jeff, but once she did, she was replying sarcastically back at him, treating him like a trusted older brother. It was so great to see Nicole open up and feel comfortable in our home.

CHAPTER 14

WHIRLWIND ADOPTION

One afternoon while the kids were at school and Jeff was at work, I came down to the kitchen to make some lunch where I found Nicole. "How you doing today?" I asked.

"I'm okay, haven't puked today so that's good," Nicole replied jokingly. Then she paused. "Do you know what I wish?" Nicole asked out of the blue.

"What?" I responded.

"I wish I knew a family who loved me that would adopt my baby," Nicole said this as she lovingly rubbed her hand over her belly.

I wasn't sure what to say at first. *Did I hear her right?* I didn't have much time to think before saying, "Well . . . we love you and we would adopt your baby if you wanted." I hadn't anticipated her response.

"Really," she cried out excitedly, "you would want my baby?"

I looked at her in shock, my mouth wide open. "Of course, if you felt like that's what you wanted, we would be honored to adopt her. Why don't you take a few days to see how it feels and I will let Jeff know that you are think-ing about this." Nicole smiled as I wrapped her up in a big hug. I couldn't believe how much I loved her in such a short amount of time.

As Nicole headed up to her room, I rushed to grab my phone to call Jeff at work. I usually didn't like to bug him at work, but this conversation couldn't wait. I anxiously paced as the phone rang, hoping he would answer the phone.

"Hey, what's up?" Jeff answered happily.

"Umm . . . I have some big news, can you talk?" I talked quickly.

"Yes, what's going on?" Jeff replied.

"Nicole just told me that she is entertaining the thought of having us adopt her baby . . . what do you think?" I held my breath as I waited for his response.

"Wow, really? That would be amazing." I was thrilled that we were on the same page.

"Of course I told her that there was no pressure and if she changed her mind, we would still be there to support her, but it's an option we need to prepare for." Jeff and I chatted a little longer before he needed to get back to work. I couldn't contain my excitement and waited for Nicole to talk to us again.

Two days later and many prayers from Nicole, she asked Jeff and I if we would adopt her little girl. Jeff was just as excited as I had been when I first heard the news. Jeff and I excitedly gathered our four sweet little kids down to talk about what was going on. They had all accepted Nicole in our home as family and liked to call her their big sister, which made my heart swell with pride. At this time, Landan was eight, Taylor was seven, Callen was four and Carter was three. All the kids gathered on our deep brown couch in the family room for the discussion we were about to have.

"So, how's everyone doing?" I started, watching the wiggly little children in front of me try their best to listen.

"Good!" they all responded while they smiled in anticipation for whatever we were going to tell them.

"You know Nicole has a baby in her tummy?" We had talked to the kids about this when Nicole moved in and told them why she was feeling sick and tired all the time.

"Yes," Landan responded happily, while Taylor nodded. Both the boys were little and weren't really paying attention. They were more distracted by poking each other than what I was saying.

"So, Nicole asked us if we would adopt her baby and we aren't sure yet if that will happen, but we are thinking about making it happen. So . . . you would all have a new baby sister. What do you think of that?"

Landan and Taylor squealed in delight. "Really? A baby sister?" Landan almost shouted.

"I can't wait to hold her," Taylor added.

Callen and Carter were off the couch playing by that point, not interested in any more additions to our family. "Hey, boys! What do you think about having a new baby sister?"

They both stopped for a brief moment and looked at me, gave me matching grins, then went back to playing. I assumed their smiles were a good sign.

Throughout the next few weeks, Landan and Taylor asked questions about the baby and were getting excited to be able to be big sisters again.

Jeff and I felt so blessed to welcome another child into our home. We hired an adoption attorney, got our background check done all in record time (three weeks) and were all ready before the baby arrived.

Our baby girl, Avery, was born in June 2012, not long after we finalized our part of the adoption. Nicole lived with us for a week before she signed the papers to relinquish her rights. It was one of the most bittersweet moments of my life. We were so thankful to be able to adopt this sweet, precious baby, but we were so sad for this sweet girl who blessed us with such an incredible gift of our fifth child.

We felt so incredibly blessed. God knew that we all needed each other.

Avery's birth mom was such a wonderful addition to our family. Even though she moved out not long after she had Avery, Nicole lived only ten minutes away. We saw her at least once a week and she created such a sweet bond with Avery and all our other children. I was so grateful that our daughter would grow up knowing her birth mom so well. I would get so overwhelmed when I told our adoption story because I knew that it was completely guided by God. We knew that our prayers were heard and everything was orchestrated by God's hands.

After such a whirlwind adoption and adding another baby—and an older girl—to our family, it seemed like things were a little more calm for a while. My heart was healing so well and I felt some restored energy as my body healed. I truly thought heart surgery was the final step to feeling good.

Day by day I was getting stronger. I could tell such a difference in my health. My energy was restored and I felt quite amazing. With renewed health, I decided I needed to start exercising once again. CrossFit was the first thing on my mind and I was anxious to start up again. It was hard and I took it very easy to begin with, lifting light weights and doing half the workout at first. I felt so weak but I knew I had to start slow.

Awful migraines were triggered again; every time I went to CrossFit, I had the worst migraine. But I wasn't going to let it stop me. I felt like my body just had to get used to exercise without a hole in my heart. Finally, after two weeks of consistent exercise, I was feeling better. Slowly I added more weight, ran farther and was making progress. I felt so blessed. What a journey I had been on. I was so thankful to be able to exercise and take care of my home and family once again.

Not long after we adopted our daughter and felt like we were getting on a good schedule with our newborn, I went to get some dental work done. My teeth had always been very bad and it seemed like I was constantly getting cavities filled or root canals done, which I always hated. After having heart surgery, I had to be on antibiotics when getting dental work done so an infection in my mouth wouldn't travel to my heart. The dental work went well and I went home to start my antibiotics.

The antibiotic given to me made me so sick, but the dentist told me to keep taking it so my heart would not get infected. Obeying the dentist and not knowing any better, I continued the antibiotics. By the end of ten days on the meds, I had vertigo so bad I could hardly walk. It was terrible. The most terrible thing about it was that my vertigo didn't go away after I stopped taking the antibiotics. It was one of the most frustrating symptoms I had ever experienced!

Not only was I having vertigo, but I was losing my memory and had major brain fog. I had always had an incredible memory; I could remember people's names and where I knew them from. I had memories from my childhood, but gradually, as my kids would ask me about my life when I was little, I couldn't remember much. If I met a new person, I would immediately forget their name. It was embarrassing and I was becoming more of a hermit. I didn't want to be around other people, not even my friends.

Some of my good friends from college, Sandi and Renee, would get together and they would tell stories of things we did. I would nod my head and laugh at the memories they were sharing and was concerned that a lot of my memories were lost. At least I had my friends to remind me of the fun we had and they could help me remember.

There were times when the vertigo went away and I was able to start driving again. One day I was driving my car with all of my children in it. My husband had told me to follow him home because he was driving a car that could possibly break down and he didn't want to be stranded if it did (he owned a car dealership and was always driving different cars). I agreed to follow him and hopped in the car. We were on the road our house was on and all of a sudden, I was very confused and didn't know where I was or where I was going. I didn't want to freak out my kids, so I tried to stay calm. Nothing looked familiar around me and I was starting to panic. I'm not sure why, but in my head, something was telling me to follow the car in front of me that I didn't recognize. I know that God was guiding me that day. My brain had stopped working, but I followed the car in front of me and not very much longer we were home in our driveway. I told Jeff what had happened and we kind of laughed about it, but it really scared me. This kind of thing happened now and then and when it would happen, I would pull over and call Jeff to tell him I was lost. It never took very long for me to remember where I was and I was able to find my way to the destination.

As if vertigo wasn't bad enough, depression and anxiety were consuming me. I had never felt so low and helpless in my life. Every time my health seemed to be improving, something happened to knock me back down in bed. I didn't know what to do. I didn't know what doctor to go to next. I basically had a specialist for every part of my body, but no one could look at the whole picture and figure out what was going on. I felt like I would never be able to find an answer to all my problems. I could not accept that I was a sick person and this was my life. It was getting harder and harder to stay positive.

CHAPTER 15

DONE WITH DOCTORS

I knew there were still many things wrong with me and I still went to countless doctors to try and find more solutions to the odd symptoms that plagued my everyday life. But I never got any new answers; in fact, the list of people in white coats who thought I was lying, attention-seeking, or downright crazy kept getting bigger.

That's when I made a decision: I was feeling decent enough now that I was done with doctors. Instead, I decided to take my husband's advice and indulge in some much-needed self-care. Jeff encouraged me to get a massage from my friend, Juanique. By then, it was the height of summer and I sat in my car in front of Juanique's beautiful new house with the A/C pumping full blast. The sun beat down on the windshield, blinding me as I gathered the physical strength to go knock on the door of where she ran her massage business in her home.

After I made my way up to her front porch, it only took seconds for Juanique to open the door. There stood my friend, whom I'd only known for about six months but we clicked immediately after meeting at church. It felt like I knew her way longer. She was wearing her usual light-colored clothes that accented her beautiful long brown hair. She wrapped me up in a warm hug. "I'm so glad you are here!" she exclaimed, her dark brown eyes sparkling from her soft, round face. "Come in."

It had been a few months since I'd seen her, but it was easy for me to feel relaxed and welcome in Juanique's beautiful, clean home. She led me into the side room that housed her massage table and I enjoyed the way the summer light streamed in through tall, gleaming window panes. *I sure hope this will make me feel better, at least for a little while.*

"So," Juanique began as she sat me down and took my purse, hanging it on a decorative little knob by the door. "I thought, after your massage, I could do some muscle testing on you, to see if your body can tell me what's going on."

I gave her a funny look, confused. I had no idea what muscle testing was and even though I hadn't known her very long, I trusted her completely and literally having nothing to lose at that point, I replied, "Sure. Why not?"

After an amazing massage, Juanique asked me to hold out my arm. I did, then she began to ask my body questions, to see what would come up. If the answer was yes to the question asked, my arm would hold strong, but if the answer was no, my arm would fall. Fascinated and a little perturbed, I silently observed this new technique.

This is a little weird, I thought, *but I don't see the harm in trying something new. The medical community has failed me. I'm all out of other options.*

I was impressed when Juanique said, "So, do you have an injury in the back of your ankle on your right leg?"

"Yes, I injured my Achilles tendon pretty badly when I was young," I replied.

"That makes sense," Juanique said as she continued asking questions. I was shocked with how accurate her findings were; I had never told her about that.

Juanique caught my eye and her face got very serious. "Well, Brita, I can tell that there's something else going on with you, but I just can't figure it out. I'm sure you're tired of having people tell you that. But trust me: I believe you really need to go see a woman I know named Dr. Sucher. She is a Naturopath and has helped a lot of my clients when they haven't been able to find out why they feel so bad. I really think she could help you."

I couldn't help but frown as I stood up and reached for my bag. "That's very kind, Juanique, but . . ." I faded off, not wanting to explain to her all the reasons why I would not be going to another doctor. But, when she wrote the doctor's contact information on a little piece of paper, I found myself accepting it nonetheless. After seeing Juanique "work her magic" with massage and muscle testing, I felt I owed it to myself and Juanique, to make one last appointment. I promised her I would call Dr. Sucher.

It seemed as though the timing had been divinely orchestrated: I found out that it usually took months to get in with Dr. Sucher, but there was a cancellation just a few days after Juanique gave me her number. So I took the opening. On the day of the appointment, I really didn't want to go; I felt like my whole married life had been spent being told bad things in doctors' offices and I had made the choice to not put myself in another painful situation yet again.

But it was too late to cancel without having to pay for the missed appointment and I didn't like to waste money. So Jeff took me to the appointment. As we drove, I tried to push aside my doubts and my bad attitude. Instead, I concentrated on how safe and grounded my husband made me feel when he was with me. *Like gravity.* He was always such an amazing support to me. I glanced sideways at him as we turned onto University Parkway and I couldn't stop the sadness from rushing into my heart. Was I really going to put him through another fruitless doctor's appointment? I couldn't bear to drag him from place to place, leaving me more discouraged than when we arrived.

"I don't want to go to another doctor. I don't want to be here," I said dejectedly as we entered the clean, small lobby.

Tenderly squeezing my hand, Jeff responded, "I know, but maybe this one will help."

As I looked up at him, his signature smile melted me on the spot like it always did, but stubborn ice remained around my heart, protecting me from further disappointment. I didn't smile back.

In fact, for some reason, that afternoon, my husband's constant positivity made anger spark in my chest. How dare he be so happy when I had been suffering for so long? No one could really help me, but he kept up his insistent, annoying string of hope. Right then, I couldn't stand it. I pulled my hand away from Jeff's and folded my arms. I swallowed my rage as I shuffled to the reception desk, wallowing in my bitter self-pity.

After checking in, I took a seat once more, barely noticing the nice, quaint furniture. Strong essential oils wafted through the air, bringing back memories of when I'd tried a regimented routine that turned out to be another failed attempt to get me better.

"Mrs. Peterson," said a nurse in the doorway, bringing my mind back to the present. She led us back to an exam room and shortly afterward, Dr. Sucher entered. Right away, the short, friendly lady seemed quite interested in my health. In fact, her genuine questions made me feel a bit better right away.

"So," Dr. Sucher said, leaning toward me with an energized tone. "Tell me more about what's going on."

"Well, I've been to a ton of different doctors," I replied as I started pulling out my most recent blood work and other test results for her to look at. I had been collecting all of my test results in a red binder that I took to the appointment. I continued at a rapid pace, "I basically have a different specialist for every part of my body, but nobody can figure out why I still feel terrible. I've been diagnosed with celiac disease, Hashimoto's, interstitial cystitis and fibromyalgia. I had a hole in my heart repaired and so many other things over the last four years. I eat healthy and yet I still feel terrible."

I paused for a moment, worried she would stop listening. Usually this was the point when other doctors' attention had waned, but when I cautiously met Dr. Sucher's gaze, she merely nodded for me to continue.

"I don't know if all of this is related, but I've had weird internal itching," I shared. "It feels like I have tiny bugs crawling all over the inside of my body, along with daily headaches and lots of migraines, more than I would like." I looked at her with all of the frustration I had been feeling. "I am so exhausted all the time . . . I just want to take care of my children and live a normal, active life . . . but . . ."

Sudden emotion clogged my throat and I found myself weeping in yet another exam room. It was always so hard to list all of my symptoms over and over to new people. *How do you explain to someone that you don't feel good all the time?* It wasn't just a symptom, it was a feeling of *yuck* every single day.

Jeff rubbed my back in encouragement to keep going, but I was so tired of trying to explain what was going on with me. I didn't have the energy to pull away from his touch once more, but I wanted to.

Dr. Sucher waited for a moment, then reached toward the counter to hand me several tissues. "Okay, Brita," she began, her tone low and comforting. "This is all very interesting. Is there anything else you'd like to share?" She jotted down notes on a small pad of paper in her lap.

Once I could control my crying, I heaved in a shaky breath. "I am *so* tired," I explained again as I grabbed more tissues. "You have to understand, I used to be an athlete. I have run a half marathon; I have always been at my best when I'm busy. But now I can hardly walk to the bathroom without getting exhausted. I feel like I have the flu all the time. Oh and my body always aches. I literally hurt all over. I get these weird tremors in my legs sometimes.

Those are really annoying. The worst thing I think is that I'm not happy like I used to be. I feel like a different person; I'm sad all the time."

I looked into the doctor's compassionate eyes and instead of being stumped, she looked intrigued. It was a look I hadn't seen in a doctor's eyes in quite some time.

At the end of the appointment, Dr. Sucher looked at me and said confidently, "With everything you have told me, I am eighty percent sure I know what's wrong with you."

I snapped my attention to Jeff briefly, my eyes wide. ". . . Really?" I asked, my voice coming out in a whisper. Was she going to tell me something new, something that had a treatment plan, or even a cure?

Dr. Sucher nodded. "I'm almost positive you have Lyme disease."

My mouth fell completely open. "So . . . what does that mean?" I managed, still in shock. "What is Lyme disease?" It was an illness I had heard of but knew nothing about. So many questions were popping up in my head and suddenly I was very scared.

The doctor reassured me, "Let's not get ahead of ourselves, Brita. I want to run some blood work to check some more things out, things that the other doctors haven't looked at."

"Okay," I began, bewildered. I couldn't help but add sarcastically, "Although I think I've had every blood test run that's possible." I was joking, even though all I wanted to do was roll up in a ball and cry my eyes out. *Are you kidding me? How can I have yet another disease?*

Dr. Sucher gave me a warm smile. "There are plenty of tests they *haven't* run, Brita. Thanks for bringing this binder with all of these tests in it; it's been very helpful to see what you have and have not had done. I know I don't know you well just yet, but believe me: I'm going to figure out why you feel so awful all the time. I am confident I can help you."

The sarcastic smirk fell off of my face. *Did I hear that right?* Those were refreshing words I never expected to hear. The tears flowed again and I could hardly speak. This time, my tears had a glimmer of hope. A part of me wanted to jump up to hug the doctor, but my overwhelming fatigue kept me squished in the comfy chair.

I snuck a glance over at Jeff, who had been sitting quietly by my side through the long appointment. Although he was quiet, his love spoke so loud to me. Something softened just then: the level of anger and rage that I had been experiencing suddenly dissipated. I knew in that moment that Jeff would continue to love me through the bumps and turns that were ahead of us. I didn't feel deserving of a man so incredible and patient.

Even though I had been a jerk earlier when we were driving to the appointment, I knew he understood. It meant the world to me that he could come to Dr. Sucher, because I hated going to the doctor alone. It was perfect that I had actually gotten good news for a change this time around.

When I was sent to get my blood drawn, the phlebotomist filled more vials than usual from me. She joked that they were taking all of my blood. *Fine. Take it all if it will help this time around.* I wasn't surprised at how negative my thoughts were because that was becoming more normal for me. However, my eyes grew wide with surprise as I counted vial after vial of my thick, dark blood.

They really are taking it all.

After getting bandaged up, I had to go home, sit and wait. A few weeks later, I returned to Dr. Sucher's office. She shared the news with me: not only did I have Lyme disease, but also a co-infection called mycoplasma. In addition, my adrenal glands were close to failing. My kidneys, pancreas and liver were hardly functioning at all. When Dr. Sucher sat down with me, I saw pure concern for my health and well-being in her gaze.

"The only other patient I have that is more complicated than you has cancer," she said honestly.

I was so relieved that I didn't have cancer, but I was devastated that my body was so sick. *No wonder I felt like crap all the time!* No wonder it felt like my body was shutting down, because we now had the test results to prove that it really was. Things could always be worse, but knowing that I was in such a bad state of health was devastating.

This new diagnosis could explain so many things. It was terribly daunting. The doctor then affirmed what I had been most afraid of: there was no cure for Lyme disease. I felt myself fighting the acceptance of that fact. I didn't want to.

Without wasting any time, I began a Lyme protocol that Dr. Sucher thought could help me at least begin to feel better. Some of these included many different antibiotics, along with tons of supplements and probiotics to fight my newfound illnesses.

What I soon discovered was that the antibiotics made me even sicker. I felt like I had a bad case of the flu for a good week or two when I would start each batch of antibiotics. This was called herxing, which meant the medicine was killing off the bad bacteria in my body. While that was good, as my body detoxed, I got very sick. My poor husband picked up all my slack, taking care of the kids, feeding them dinner and everything else, while working full-time. I was barely surviving.

I called Kirsti to vent my frustrations. "Hey sis, you busy?" I tried to sound happy, but she knew me well enough to hear my voice breaking.

"What's going on?" Kirsti got straight to the point.

I started crying and she sat there in silence with me for a few minutes while I tried to pull myself together. "I can't do this anymore. I'm so tired of being sick. I feel awful all the time and I don't know why I can't get better. Everything I try doesn't work. I am so frustrated. I'm sorry to call and cry to you but I just need to vent to someone." We had talked earlier in the week about my Lyme disease diagnosis; I always updated her on what was going on.

"It's okay, you can always call me," Kirsti reassured me.

My sister had become one of my lifelines. I had Jeff who was always there and my parents, but I didn't like to let them know how bad I was feeling. Since Kirsti had dealt with some depression, I knew she could understand what I was going through.

We talked for a while and eventually Kirsti had me laughing, which was something I always loved about her. Suddenly the conversation wasn't so heavy and an idea popped into my head, out of the blue. For a split second, I worried about bringing it up, since it was a sensitive subject. I didn't want to trigger Kirsti's depression or cause her more angst.

I'm not sure why it even entered my head, since we were laughing and joking, trying to get my mind off my sadness. But the thought had come on strong and it wasn't going away. I shared with her, knowing she'd listen to anything, even if it was hard to say out loud.

"This is a weird question," I blurted, "but do you think we were . . . ummm . . ." I swallowed hard. ". . . sexually abused . . . maybe when we were little or something?"

I waited silently, holding my breath, not knowing how she would react to such a question. I was surprised when she said quietly, "You know, I always wondered that too."

"Really?" I shot back. "Why do you think that?"

"I don't know, I've just always wondered, with the depression we have dealt with. We grew up in a home with supportive parents and there is no reason we should be so depressed."

We talked about it a little longer. There were other things that had made me question this but since I didn't have any memories of anyone hurting me in that way, I didn't think much more about it. It was nice being able to open up to Kirsti; it always helped me feel a little better.

One night after Jeff got the kids in bed, he lay by me. It was our special time together and as usual he gestured to me and said, "Give me a foot." He had taken to rubbing my feet almost every night while I cried to him. That night was no different.

"Jeff, I can't do this anymore. I feel terrible." As soon as the tears started, I couldn't make them stop. "I feel like such an awful mom! I can't even get out of bed to pick them up from school. Why have I been sick for so long? I'm *so* tired of being sick. I don't have any friends and I feel like I've been too needy for too long."

I cried some more. I knew I still had wonderful friends that continued to help me, but while their lives were moving forward, mine was on perpetual repeat of the same sad story.

"I know it sucks, but you are a great mom," Jeff insisted compassionately. "You can't help that all these things are making you sick. You are doing your best. And you have so many friends that love you. I know you feel alone, but you aren't. And I love you so much and so do the kids."

That should have cheered me up, but it didn't. I tried so hard to stay positive, but everyone around me had no idea the suffering I was experiencing. I didn't want anyone—even Jeff—knowing what was really going on because I knew they wouldn't understand. It would just make me more mad that they couldn't get it. The darkness was settling in all around me and it felt like I might suffocate.

Luckily not too long after Jeff started rubbing my feet, my medication kicked in. It made me drowsy and, relieved, I fell into a deep sleep.

Waking up the next morning didn't bring rest, but after the kids and Jeff left for the day, I went into my solitary routine, trying to find some comfort while I was alone and combatting a new, unseen enemy. I watched movies and played card games on my phone to keep my mind busy. I fought as hard as I could to keep my mind from spiraling into the deep, ugly darkness that was always just one thought away.

CHAPTER 16

BROKEN

If Jeff isn't home soon, I'm going to be late!

I fumed on the inside while I angrily paced the kitchen. Every time I whipped around to look at the clock, my temper raged higher. He knew that I hated being late and now I wasn't going to make it to Avery's school meeting because of him.

"Eat your dinner!" I snapped over my shoulder at the kids, who were gathered around the table. *"Now!"*

Finally, I saw him coming up the driveway. The second he got in the door, I glared at him.

"Sorry I'm late," Jeff began, but I already ripped the Mustang keys out of his hand.

"Love you all," I said dryly as I stormed out the door, not even looking back at my family.

Lately, despite every medication and every tool I tried, my emotions were just out of control. Little things were always a big deal. If something changed in my schedule, I would freak out and tonight was no exception. As I pulled out of the driveway, annoyance crept into my head, irritated that yet again I'd gotten upset over such a small thing. I was getting tired of apologizing to Jeff and the kids for losing my temper over the dumbest situations. Being angry all the time was dragging me down, but I felt so out of control all of the time and there was nothing I could do about it. On top of always being angry, my anxiety was heightened and it was hard for me to do simple tasks.

Now, on my own with nothing between me and the power behind our car's steering wheel, I at least felt a little bit of control. The light turned green and I accelerated, loving the speed and power of the convertible. I didn't even want to go to this meeting, but I had to try and pull myself together so I could pretend that everything was fine for an hour in front of the other parents.

As I sped up, my mind craved more speed. I was usually a cautious driver, having never gotten a speeding ticket, but tonight I felt careless. That feeling danced across my skin and down to my fingertips, frightening me. It was almost as if I wasn't in control as my foot plunged harder on the gas pedal. A smile split across my face as the car effortlessly flew down the street. My brain was losing control. All of a sudden I had the urge to accelerate until the pedal hit the floor mat.

Then I could slam right into that next telephone pole. I was surprised at the thought, but in a way it seemed nice. *Maybe if I just crash, this can be done with. Yes . . . this is it. Here I go.*

Before I could get up to speed, I spotted flashing police lights down the road. Disappointment filled me as I was forced to slow down with the rest of traffic. There was clearly an accident of some kind ahead. Cautiously, I went around the police cars, then noticed a car wrapped around a telephone pole. Something clicked in my brain. As soon as I was away from the crash, I pulled over and started crying hysterically.

Oh my gosh! What is wrong with me? I said a prayer for the people involved in the accident that somehow they would be okay, even though I didn't think anyone could have survived that. Gripping the wheel tightly, with tears soaking the front of my jacket, I gathered a deep, shaky breath and turned my fury toward God.

"What is wrong with me?" I shouted at my windshield. "How can You let me have these kinds of thoughts? I don't want to die. I have to be here to take care of my sweet kids." A sob broke through as fresh tears blinded me. "I love them so much. I would never want to leave them. But I feel so alone . . . are You even there? Can You hear me? Can You hear me?" I yelled it again, hoping to hear some sort of response but the silence was deafening.

For all the years of my life, when I had prayed to a God I loved, I always felt some kind of peace after baring my soul. But sitting on the side of the road that night, I only found myself surrounded with crushing silence. There was no comfort and I began to crumble to pieces when my eyes drifted to my phone. The name of my good friend JB entered my head. I knew that if I wanted to make it through the rest of the night, I had to call her right away.

"JB . . . are you home?" was all I could get out before I couldn't talk through the tears.

Somehow I made it to her house and opened up about all of my dark thoughts and feelings. It was embarrassing to admit what I almost did to myself. Had I not seen that accident that had been so eerily similar to my own plans, I might have really done something stupid. As much as I felt bad for the people in that car, I was so grateful that seeing them had snapped me out of those awful thoughts. After a couple hours of crying and talking in my car with JB in the passenger seat, I felt much better. Glancing out the windshield, I realized it had gotten very dark and my only option was to head back home. I didn't make it to that meeting after all.

Over the next few months, my suicidal feelings were still present. They surfaced in new forms at different times, wreaking havoc on my emotions and impeding my ability to care for my family. I thought back to the time in college when I had accidentally cut my wrist on that barbed wire fence. Glancing down at my arm one afternoon before I had to get the kids from school, I saw only the faded remains of a scar from my stitches.

I was such a different person back when I was only nineteen years old. I'd given that ER nurse the weirdest look when she'd asked me about whether I'd harmed myself that night. I never had experienced depression, much less suicidal thoughts. In those days, I was so happy and full of life. But now, I could hardly find a happy thought in my head. I missed the old me. *Will I ever be myself again?*

One night late into winter, when frigid temperatures had settled into the valley, I shivered as my five-year-old cried out down the hall. She was having a hard time staying asleep lately and needed me to get up often to soothe her back into the comfort of her dreams. But I groaned against the aspect of getting out of my warm bed. Heaviness lay on me that had nothing to do with the thick blanket on my body or the tall piles of overwhelming snow outside. I could barely find the motivation to rise and stumble sleepily into Avery's room to gather her in my arms.

When I was able to crawl back into bed, sleep found me once more until my alarm blared in my ears mere hours later. Slamming my hand down against the button to shut it off, I nudged Jeff and murmured for him to wake up the kids for school. Even though I'd gone to bed early the night before, I still felt exhausted. I needed him to tackle the morning's tasks for me.

Each of my five children came to give me a warm hug before they left for school as I still laid in my comfy bed. It was now the place I never wanted to leave. After the house emptied, I felt so guilty for being happy that they were all gone. I still loved my entire family, but no matter how many doctors I saw or procedures I had or medications I took or diagnoses I received, I never had the energy to take care of anyone. Until I had to pick up my kids from school, I had a small window of alone time and I was so ashamed to feel relieved.

As I struggled to lift my head off the soft pillow a few hours later, I winced in pain. Tears of anger filled my eyes. I was so exasperated that my body had completely betrayed me. As I struggled to walk the ten steps to the bathroom, my mind was flooded with memories of who I used to be. It was almost comical that I could hardly walk ten easy steps when I had run a half marathon five years ago.

You used to be a dancer, Brita! I shamefully reminded myself as I flicked on the light switch. *And a singer! Remember the days when you played competitive basketball? Fast-pitch softball? Remember when you ran track and made it to state?*

The weight on my shoulders pressed down further, burying me in self-pity that I couldn't escape and didn't even bother denying. Back when I played soccer, I would get carded for slide-tackling my opponents. I used to be fierce. I used to be a fighter. There wasn't anything that would take me out of a game. *Now look at me: I can hardly walk to the bathroom, let alone take care of my children. I'm a complete failure.*

This wasn't how my life was supposed to be. I glanced up at the bathroom mirror and blinked in terror at my reflection. I didn't even recognize myself. The person before me could no longer fit in the cute size-six jeans that I loved. I certainly didn't feel pretty and I definitely felt sorry for anyone that had to be around me.

That afternoon, I was somehow able to find the energy to pick up my kids from school. It made me happy I could at least do that, but as I glanced at my children in the rear view mirror, I wondered what they really thought of me. When we made it home from picking everyone up, I crawled back into bed, distracting myself with another movie. As soon as Jeff got home, I asked him to take the kids out for dinner, because I'd been unable to prepare a meal yet again for them that night. My amazing husband just smiled at me, kissed me gently and happily took the kids out to eat.

The house was once again empty and my brokenness finally consumed me completely. I couldn't stop crying. I was so far from the girl I used to be and this shattered person that I was, she was nothing I recognized.

I needed to do something to feel better and decided that a hot bath was just what I needed. Running the tub, I let the soothing sound of water rush over me, begging for some kind of relief to enter my mind. After pouring in some epsom salt, I climbed in and lay my head back against the hard, cold porcelain of the tub.

Please, God, I begged as the steam rose around me, *heal my body. Take away my pain and suffering. I promise I'll serve and take care of everyone around me if I can just feel good enough to get out of bed. Why won't You help me?*

Even though I didn't feel close to God at all, I thought that He loved me. Didn't I have enough faith all of these years? Couldn't He afford me this one miracle so my family could have the loving mother and wife they deserved? I knew that my vibrant, giving husband should have a healthy partner he didn't have to take care of every day. I knew my children would be better off if they had a mom who could be with them when they needed her. But my body was shutting down. All hope was lost.

With numb hands and a heavy heart, I slowly scrubbed my face with soap. After there were plenty of bubbles, I bent forward with my face in the water to rinse it off. It didn't take long, but I decided to not raise my head. I stayed under the water with my eyes closed, tears suddenly flooding the bathtub.

This was it. All I had to do was stay there. Soon, I could be singing with angels or dancing in hell, I didn't care which one. My breath was running out. The darkness kept my head under, like the devil himself was pulling me down.

CHAPTER 17

GET ME OFF THIS ROLLERCOASTER

Something made me raise my head. I don't know what it was, but an unexpected force had me pulling my face out of the water, where I gasped and sputtered for air. Shaking droplets off of my cheeks and across the wood floor in the bathroom, I marveled at the power that had suddenly told me to breathe. In that moment I felt energy race into my veins as I immediately climbed out of the tub and pulled the plug. My heart was racing as I wrapped a towel around my shaking body and ran into my bedroom.

What the heck just happened? Was that my prayer being answered . . . after all this time, did I get an answer from God about whether I should still be alive or not?

Collapsing against my cool pillows, I silently vowed to not take a bath again for a long time. I knew I couldn't survive like this much longer and said another fervent prayer for strength. Clearly, whatever force had stopped me from drowning myself felt that I still needed to be here. I had to dig deep, find what was left of the fighter in me and tell her to *get up*. This wasn't over, even if every challenge so far seemed like an insurmountable wall. Whatever was wrong with me, I couldn't let it defeat me in such a way that I'd almost embraced it in that warm, sudsy water. I had to not give up.

Time went by and I made every effort I could to be there for my family. I had some good days and pushed myself to the limits during them, doing everything with my kids and Jeff with my scraps of energy. I made it to cheer competitions, dance recitals, basketball games and even to the horse arena. Whenever I could, I pushed through the pain and the weight of the depression.

A year and a half passed and I continued my fight against Lyme disease and every other co-infection that came with it. Eventually, I hit a plateau with Dr. Sucher. We did everything we could together to make strides forward with my treatment, despite the cost and the time. Eventually, Jeff and I found a place in Idaho called The West Clinic, where they offered powerful

IV vitamin treatments. I tried several different options with them, including ozone therapy, which involved drawing some of my blood, running it through an ozone machine to help purify it, then putting it back in my body.

For over another year that made a big difference, despite having to travel back and forth to Idaho. I was lucky to have family nearby whom I could stay with after getting my treatments. Slowly, I began to grow new sparks of hope. These new things were helping and when a clinic was opened in Salt Lake, I immediately was excited to go there instead to avoid such a long drive. My new doctor, Dr. Watson, was amazing at digging to see what was going on with me. If my health stopped improving, she would run more tests, continuing to find what was plaguing my body so I could continue to heal. Dr. Watson was a very important doctor in my healing journey. Her clinic offered many healing modalities, medical and holistic, that continued to improve my health. At least she was constantly trying anything she could to help me feel better, even though my body was still struggling. The daily treatments were not only rough on my body but I started getting severe anxiety about having to get poked everyday for the IVs. Dr. Watson suggested I get a PICC line placed to make things easier for me. I knew it would help me calm down since I wouldn't be constantly pricked with needles every time I had to get a treatment.

One afternoon, I opened the front door to find a package waiting for me. It was covered in stickers with Japanese on them and my heart leapt. A good friend of mine who was a roommate in college lived in Japan at that time. Becky often sent me things in the mail to lift my spirits through my health struggles.

Inside I found a lovely necklace. Along with it was a booklet with the company name *The Nozomi Project*. Reading on, I learned that they made jewelry out of broken pottery from the tsunami that hit the country recently. My eyes filled with tears as I read on:

"Holding Hope. This necklace is made from broken pottery in Ishinomaki, Japan by a community of women who survived the 2011 tsunami. Wear it as a reminder of beauty in brokenness. #bebrokenwithus"

Those words touched me and I put the necklace on right away. Becky had also written me a sweet note of her own, encouraging me like she always did. I glanced at the clock on my kitchen wall and knew that I should wait until later in the evening to call her at a decent time on the other side of the world so I could properly thank her for such a beautiful and thoughtful gift.

Whenever I wore that necklace, it gave me hope that I could be polished through my trials. As I continued to do everything I could to get better, it served as a reminder that something beautiful could come out of all of this despair. Wearing a piece of brokenness on my own broken body felt as if I was embracing a new magical power, along with the new treatments. I was seeing small amounts of improvements and the good days started to outweigh the bad ones. There was hope again.

CHAPTER 18

REMISSION

"Brita, is that you?"

I turned away from the grocery store shelf full of little pill bottles when I heard my name. It was rare for me to be shopping, but this health store was close by and I needed some vitamin D. I grinned in surprise when I saw my friend Juanique, the massage therapist who had introduced me to Dr. Sucher, smiling down at me. She leaned in for a hug, wrapping her long, lanky arms around me and I squeezed her back. We hadn't spoken much in the last couple of years since she'd moved out of state, so it was a wonderful surprise to see her that afternoon.

Juanique pulled back, staring into my eyes with a look of concern. "How are you?" she asked quietly.

"Well . . ." I began slowly. "I'm hanging in there, I guess." She knew a little bit about what I'd faced in my life, but lately so many ups and downs had occurred that I didn't want to begin explaining them. "I'm doing okay," I added, smiling more brightly. This woman always had such a warmth about her that I couldn't help but feel better.

"Are you still struggling?" Juanique questioned, getting right to the point.

"Yes," I sighed as I confessed the real truth. "I haven't been doing very well. My depression has been terrible and my body is so sick. I just can't get better and I'm so frustrated. Everything I try seems so temporary."

Juanique nodded as if she completely understood. Even though I hadn't seen her lately, it was as if no time had passed at all when we spoke. "Well, I have some good news," she began happily. "Since we got back to Utah, we opened up a clinic behind my mother's apothecary business. Brita, we have *two* hyperbaric oxygen machines in there!"

I raised my eyebrows, intrigued. I had heard of these machines helping people with all kinds of ailments, but never thought it would be the right fit for me. If I had cancer, maybe, or an infection that wouldn't go away, it would make sense since that was what hyperbaric machines were typically used for.

"I keep thinking of you and want you to come try one out," Juanique insisted, putting an encouraging hand on my arm. "I will text you a link to some research about the HBOT—that's the short name for it. Let me know if you want to come in for some treatments. We also have some other things that I really think can help you."

When I met Juanique's cheerful gaze, I felt the overflow of positive energy that she always exuded. I was finding it really hard to come up with a reason to say no. Jeff would be incredibly supportive of any new treatments, as usual. And after all, what did I have to lose at this point? Even though I was doing okay with Dr. Watson, I wasn't making the strides forward that I had hoped.

"Okay," I caved. "What do I need to do and when can I start?"

The following week after Jeff and I had gotten all the kids to school on a crisp spring morning, we drove silently to Provo Health for my consultation. When we pulled up to the clinic it seemed too small to hold a hyperbaric chamber. After giving each other skeptical glances, my husband and I walked up to the glass doors and peered in, making sure we were in the right place.

Inside was a tiny, square shop full of oils, vitamins and supplements. A little bit of everything healthy filled every space on the walls. The bell rang when we walked in and Juanique stepped through a door in the back.

"Alright, my friend!" Juanique announced after greeting us both. She rubbed her hands together excitedly. "Let's get started!"

We began with a hair analysis that was supposed to give Juanique some clues as to what my body was lacking. She carefully pulled out a couple of my hairs from the root and put them in a machine to be read. The results wouldn't be back for a few days, so Juanique led me into a smaller room, where she placed weird boots on my feet.

"These are for foot compression therapy," she explained, "which helps the body boost immunity."

Even though the boots squeezed my feet pretty tightly, it was a relaxing therapy that I did my best to enjoy. As I closed my eyes, I couldn't help the honest skepticism that began to fill my mind. I hadn't heard of "hair analysis" or "foot compression therapy" before in my life and I had been to countless doctors over countless years. Was any of this really going to help? And where was the HBOT machine? My mind was taken back to when Juanique introduced me to muscle testing and I don't know how it was so accurate, but it worked. Juanique knew what she was doing and I had nothing to lose being here with her.

I've worn out the western medical community, I reminded myself. *It's time to be ready to try anything that can help. And I trust Juanique completely, which is more than I can say for many of my doctors.*

Before leaving the clinic, Juanique and I set up a plan for me to get forty HBOT treatments and fifteen to twenty sessions of hyperthermic ozone and carbonic acid transdermal therapy (or HOCATT). It was a bit overwhelming, but I was optimistic that I would make some progress in my health.

One week later, in early April, I went back to Provo Health to go over my hair sample analysis. Afterward, it would be time for my first HBOT. Juanique sat me down at the back of the shop and handed over a copy of the results.

"You're lacking some vitamins and minerals," she shared with me. "And you have some food sensitivities. It looks like your hormone and cardiovascular systems are struggling, too."

I was a bit surprised that a couple pieces of hair could show all of that. Even though I wasn't sure how a hair analysis worked, the details in front of me seemed to line up with the recent blood work I had done with my doctor.

Juanique set me up with some new supplements to support my body. "Are you ready?" she asked, giving me a calm smile.

I nodded. For some reason, despite the innumerable tests and therapies I'd tried already to get healthy, I was nervous for this one. I came in my comfy sweats and my favorite grey t-shirt since I would be in the chamber for an hour and a half.

When Juanique led me into the next room, I saw both machines that looked like long beds encased in clear tubes. Relief washed over me when I realized the chamber was glass that I could see through during the entire process. Juanique pulled the bed out of the chamber and had me climb on, making sure my pillow and knee pillow were comfortable.

"It might seem a little weird, but I'm going to slide you in, then close the chamber up," Juanique explained. "You will be able to hear me through a speaker and if you need anything, just talk or wave at me. The pressure dropping in the tank may hurt your ears a little. If it does, just raise your hand and we will stop to let your ears adjust. You might need to plug your nose and blow softly to help your ears clear."

I nodded, even though I was already breaking out in a sweat. My heart beat rapidly, overwhelmed by all the information being thrown at me. The HBOT machine looked like a large time capsule and I wasn't sure if I really wanted to be sealed in there.

"Also," Juanique added as she handed me an oxygen mask to wear, "would you like to watch a movie while you are in there? We have an iPad on top of the chamber if you want to watch something?"

"I'm a little nervous," I confessed with Juanique, "so no, I don't want to watch a movie. I think I will just try to sleep while I'm in here. I'm so tired."

"Perfect," Juanique said with another smile. After I slid into the tube, she shut the door tightly behind me. "We're going to start dropping the pressure," came the sound of Juanique's voice through a speaker above my head. "Let me know if you need me to slow down. I will go slow anyway, but let me know if you need anything."

I nodded and after a few minutes, everything seemed fine as silence fell and I tried to relax enough to close my eyes. Then I felt a sharp pain in my ears. "Umm, can you stop please?" I began with an edge in my voice. "My ears are killing me!"

"Of course," Juanique replied and instructed that the pressure be maintained for a moment. "Are you okay in there?" she asked.

"My ears just aren't adjusting," I said nervously.

"Plug your nose and blow softly. See if that helps," she encouraged in her calm voice.

Taking a slow, deep breath, I followed her advice. Nothing happened at first, so I tried again and finally my ears began to pop. Relief spread over me, starting at my ears and flowing down to my toes. *I can do this.* She continued to drop the pressure and even though she had to stop a few more times for me to adjust my ears, we finally arrived where I was supposed to be. Juanique checked in on me once more before I closed my eyes and fell fast asleep.

Before I knew it, I heard someone calling me awake. "Brita, it's time to come back up. You ready?"

I opened my eyes, smiled and nodded. I couldn't remember the last time I'd been able to peacefully rest for an hour and a half, in complete silence. That was a much needed nap and I was surprised how fast I had fallen asleep. After slowly bringing the pressure back up with no problems from my ears, I was guided to the HOCATT to help my body detox.

From the research that Juanique had previously sent me, I knew that this particular machine was a small sauna about the size of a person that I could sit in. It was used to increase my circulation so I could sweat out anything left in my system after the HBOT I'd just experienced.

Entering the HOCATT naked was a little weird, but I privately undressed and got into the hard plastic sauna and was completely covered before Juanique came in. She adjusted the settings for the thirty-minute treatment. I leaned my head back and relaxed as I listened to the soft yoga music that echoed peacefully around me.

Afterward, I thanked Juanique and headed over to pick up Avery from kindergarten. When we got home, I put on a movie for her and snuggled up to her as I slept again. Those sessions wiped me out, but I had a renewed sense of hope because I definitely didn't feel worse. *Maybe Juanique is right and this will be the breakthrough I need to feel like myself again.*

Over the next six weeks, I had an HBOT session five days a week and HOCATT once or twice a week. The treatments made me very tired and quite sick for the first couple of weeks, but slowly, I started feeling better after each treatment. Even though I was teased that I kept sleeping in the HBOT, I began to have more energy in the day to spend with my kids. My depression was lifting as well, which was such a relief.

My oldest daughter had a cheer competition coming up in Florida, in the middle of May. Jeff and I were planning to take our whole family so we could support Landan and also take the kids to Disney World. I was a little nervous to go on the trip, but as the time to depart got closer, I was feeling better and better. I had energy and was actually excited to go out of town with my family. That was a feeling I hadn't experienced in a long time!

We all settled in for our red-eye flight and the kids did great as excitement buzzed all around the plane cabin. Even though I was still tired, I felt like I could still go swimming at the hotel with the kids in the afternoon once we got settled in. The pool was so relaxing, surrounded by the warm Florida sun and soothing clouds. Hearing my kids' laughter was the only medicine I needed in those moments.

The next day we went to Disney World. Jeff and I decided it would be a good idea for me to get a wheelchair so I didn't overwhelm my body and it turned out to be a great choice. Jeff pushed me around as the kids walked on either side of me as we braved the crowds to experience the magic of Disney all together. My heart swelled with love when I breathed in what it felt like to be out with all of my children and my loving husband. Being able to ride the rides with them and seeing their delight was like a new beginning for me: if I could do this after just six weeks of these new treatments, imagine what I could be capable of if I kept moving forward with as much bravery and strength.

There were plenty of yummy gluten-free food options across the amusement park and the areas outside of it, so I felt I could relax even more and I was thoroughly enjoying myself. I had been so nervous to come, but now those nerves were gone and I was enjoying this time with my family.

Friday came and we went to watch Landan's cheer team compete. As she entered the stage, my eyes filled with happy tears. I glanced beside me at all my kids watching their sister and I knew these memories would continue to give me strength in the days to come. I could hardly believe I was there with enough energy to cheer and clap loudly after the performance. I felt so blessed.

Coming back home, however, I began to worry that I would need a week to recover from the trip. In the past, taking on such physical challenges always left me useless and exhausted, but guess what? This time, it didn't. I continued the HBOT treatments, making sure to throw my arms in gratitude around Juanique as soon as I saw her.

By the time my forty treatments were over, I was feeling amazing, especially when I laced up my running shoes and went for a brisk walk in the afternoon, taking the kids to the park all on my own. Dr. Watson was intrigued by my progress and how well I was doing. I told her about the HBOT and how much it was doing for me. She was so happy I was doing so well.

As fall approached and the upcoming school year began, I kept having a feeling that I should apply for some jobs. There had been so many good days recently and my anxiety and depression were getting better thanks to the HBOT and the ketamine nasal spray that Dr. Watson prescribed for me. The ketamine was a compounded nasal spray to help ease the depression. I found that I was not sinking so far down if I took the nasal spray a few times a week. It felt good to have something that worked almost immediately to relieve the little bits of depression I was still occasionally experiencing. It was such a relief to know something finally could help me feel a little more mentally stable.

I applied to a handful of jobs with some clear expectations I had for myself: *I will only work if I find a position that coincides with my kids' school schedule. It has to pay what I want and has to involve my graphic design skills that I've missed being able to use.*

It all sounded too good to be true, but three weeks later, I was surprised to find myself sitting in an interview. The position had the hours of 8:00am to 2:00pm while my kids were in school and estimated the pay I had hoped for. Because I wasn't always able to do the physical things I wanted to do, working kept my brain active and I felt like I accomplished a lot without wearing myself out. It was time for me to be creative and productive again outside of my family life, so I was thrilled when they offered me the job!

While the kids were all in full-day school, it was nice for me to have something scheduled for me to do while I was home alone, missing them. The income was really nice as well and it felt amazing to be contributing to paying down all the medical debts I had collected over the years. Getting out of debt would be such a relief, but I knew that would take time to accomplish, since we had acquired a lot of bills, trying anything and everything to help me.

I was so happy to be living again and couldn't believe I was in such a good place physically and mentally. There were so many times when I didn't think I would survive the challenges that I was facing, but now my future was looking so bright. I couldn't wait to see what was ahead of me and I was ready to face it head on.

CHAPTER 19

BEFORE I SHATTER

Feeling good emotionally and better physically was amazing. I felt like I could live like this forever if I had to. Sure, I wasn't able to do all the things I wanted to do, but it was certainly better than I'd been feeling. I was doing so well when we went to visit my parents in Oregon with the kids. They loved visiting their grandparents. We relaxed by the pool, visited my aunts, uncles and grandma. It was nice to be back where I grew up in the slow-paced little town.

After we had been there a couple days, my mom came up to me and said, "You know, Muddy Frogwater days is going on. Would you like to take the kids down there and check it out? No pressure, but it might be fun to go for a little bit."

"Sure, that sounds fun," I said and was excited to go to the little hometown festival that I hadn't attended since high school.

We drove over to Yantis Park where Muddy Frogwater was set up and as I got out of the car, the smell of deep-fried food hit me in the face. I smiled as I recognized this same smell from when I was young. It was a tiny festival with about ten small businesses, more like a farmers' market with booths of food and knick-knacks to buy. Up on the outdoor stage there was live music. It looked like a high school student out for her debut, singing her heart out to a song I didn't know. She had a nice voice and it was a fun atmosphere to be in. As we got closer to the main booth, we noticed there was a fun run. Since I was feeling really good, my mom and I signed up for the fun run. We put Avery in the stroller and the rest of the kids walked and jogged with us the whole three miles, out of the park and around the small town of Milton-Freewater, going through neighborhoods I had walked through as a teenager with my friends. I was tired but I was so happy to be doing something active again. Running was something I had missed doing so much.

As much fun as it was, my heart was racing from the hot sun and the extra exercise that my body wasn't used to. I brushed it off, proud of myself as I crossed over the finish line. We weren't fast, but we finished. I could hardly believe that I was able to do that.

After the run, we approached one of the booths and got lunch for us and the kids. I was worn out from the jog and was happy to sit and eat our food as we listened to the live music that continued, this time it was a middle-aged man and his band playing some sort of rock music. For such a small town, there was a good turnout at Muddy Frogwater and I was surprised at the handful of people I ran into that I had grown up with. It was nice catching up and hanging out with Mom. It had been so long since I could really enjoyed being out and about.

We eventually loaded up the kids and headed back to my parents' house. The energy I had started out the week with was fading a little bit but really I felt like I was on top of the world. It felt great to be living again. I might not be running half marathons, but I was out of bed enjoying myself and my family. What could be better than that? The next few days I was so tired, but it was to be expected after traveling, going for a jog and staying up late visiting with my parents. I brushed it off and knew I would have to rest and recover when I got home.

The next week I had a hard time getting up in the mornings. I didn't think much of it until, two weeks later, I was still very sluggish in the mornings. *Oh no, not this again.* It dawned on me that I might have relapsed again.

I wasn't too worried because I knew the hyperbaric chamber would get me feeling good in no time. I called Juanique and got an appointment set up. As Juanique was dropping the pressure in the chamber, I had to stop her because I was getting a very sharp pain in my nose and ears. Juanique stopped to let my ears pressurize and then tried again. This time it felt like a knife was being stabbed into my nose. "Ouch!" I yelled. "It really hurts. I don't think I can keep going."

I got out of the tank and Juanique questioned if I might have a sinus infection or something that was causing my pain. I hadn't had any symptoms, but was eager to get back to the doctor and get this figured out so I could get back in the chamber as quickly as possible. I was so disappointed since this was the only thing I knew to catapult me into remission again from this awful disease called Lyme that I was very sick of.

Back to Dr. Watson I went. She ordered more blood work and shoved a nasal swab deep in my nose to test for any sinus infections and sent me home with more supplements while we waited once more for the tests to come back.

Two weeks later, I was back, sitting in the all-too-familiar quaint little office of Dr. Watson. It was a clean but congested space, with barely enough room for a small desk. I sat in an overstuffed black chair on one side of the tiny desk, Dr. Watson on the other.

At least it was a comfy spot. So many doctors' offices had very uncomfortable chairs that I sat in while listening to frustrating or heartbreaking news, but not here. Dr. Watson made me feel relaxed and more at home. Behind her was a large window with the blinds closed. The only light coming in was from the light above us from a fluorescent light. I wasn't happy to be here again, but here I was.

"So, did you find anything?" I asked Dr. Watson in an irritated tone.

"Well," she started, "yes. You do have MARCoNS."

I sat digesting the news.

She continued, "MARCoNS is a type of staph infection that is resistant to some antibiotics. But I had your blood tested and I know what antibiotic will help you."

I stared at Dr. Watson, not wanting to believe her. I slumped down in my chair and gave her a disapproving look.

Her smile was warm and her eyes held so much compassion, I knew she wanted me to feel good and she was trying her best to help me. I wanted to be happy and joke around with her; she felt more like a friend than a doctor, but I just didn't have it in me. The depression was back and I didn't have much of a sense of humor lately.

"So, more antibiotics?" I said in disgust.

Are you kidding me? Can't I catch a break? Every time I have tests run, they come back with something new. I am so sick of being sick. Dear God, I hope this works.

"Yes and you need to be on some good probiotics and other supplements as well. I have a whole protocol for you to follow," Dr. Watson continued kindly.

Some of my grumpiness dissipated. Even though I felt the heavy weight of unhappiness that day, I was ready to do what needed to be done to help me. I was just worn out and tired of taking medicine every time I turned around.

I was hoping this was an easy fix and quick recovery, but it didn't seem like anything was that easy for me. Dr. Watson explained, "This infection is very hard to treat and it won't go away very fast. But I'm hopeful it will clear up with the nasal sprays, nebulizer treatments and the antibiotics that I will have you take."

Dr. Watson then leaned across the desk and added, "I hate to say this, but you have also relapsed with Lyme. We need to start treating that again as well."

My body stiffened with fresh shock. That unexpected news really pissed me off. "Are you kidding me?" I burst out. "Am I ever going to get better?"

Dr. Watson's next words were encouraging but I zoned out and stopped listening. She was always so positive and believed she could help, but I was having a hard time believing her. I left her office feeling discouraged and angry, with a whole bag full of items to try and I wasn't optimistic I would be feeling better soon.

I longed to be running, but instead, I was back in my bed, not only fighting the sinus infection, but Lyme disease again. The only treatment that had really helped me, I couldn't even do, since I had the sinus infection. I was so discouraged. My depression continued to creep in stronger every day and I found myself needing my ketamine spray almost every night to fight the battle with my mind. I was losing my will to keep fighting. I had already felt so broken and you would think it would be good to have windows of health, but it almost made feeling sick again much harder. The ups and downs were like a punch in the face where the bruising never has time to heal and it just keeps getting worse and worse.

I wasn't sure I could keep up this battle. I thought back to the night I almost didn't leave the tub and I shuddered. I knew I couldn't go back to that awful place in my mind. I had tried to keep most of this to myself, not sharing the news with even Jeff. I didn't want him worrying again, but I couldn't pretend to be happy anymore and even though he saw the ketamine I was taking nightly, I had reassured him it was just a precaution.

One night, I slumped in my soft, warm bed. I leaned forward, my hands becoming wet with all my new tears.

"What's wrong?" Jeff sweetly replied as he rubbed my back.

As I opened up to Jeff and told him I had relapsed and my depression was back really strong, I fell into his shoulder exhausted, feeling so defeated.

"Jeff, I can't do this anymore; everything I have tried has helped for a little bit, but then I'm back in bed crying, barely able to move my body. I have tried everything. The hyperbaric helped so much and I thought I was done being sick. Maybe I was too optimistic, but I just thought I could live the rest of my life feeling pretty good. I didn't need to feel great, but I could live okay feeling just pretty good." I lay my head on Jeff's chest as he continued to gently caress my back and I drenched his shirt with my tears.

"I don't even know what to do from here. I'm so frustrated and terrified to go back to that awful depression. I can't go back there, Jeff. I just can't."

Jeff leaned forward to give me a soft kiss on the back of the head. "I'm so sorry you are feeling bad again. You are so strong and I love you so much. I'm here for you." He wrapped me up tighter in his arms and squeezed me even closer to his chest. I felt safe there. He was always giving me encouragement and made me feel strong even though I didn't feel that way myself.

Jeff continued, "I know this is hard for you, but I know you can keep going. How about I go get your ketamine spray and see if it will help you feel a little better."

I hadn't even thought of that and was relieved Jeff had mentioned it. When I was feeling depressed, sometimes it was hard for me to know how to help myself. I felt so lucky to have an amazing man by my side. I responded, "Oh, yes that's a good idea, I think I need something to lift my mood a little tonight." I was happy the kids were in bed so they didn't have to see me breaking down.

I started inhaling the puffs one at a time, five minutes apart for five sprays. I usually only needed about three sprays but tonight I needed all the help I could get. By the fifth spray, I started feeling loopy and started laughing. "Oh no," I said slowly, "I need to go to the bathroom, can you help me walk there?" I giggled as the room seemed to be moving around me. Was it the room or in my head? I didn't know.

Jeff came around to the side of my bed, laughing as he helped me up, then he turned his back to me, lifting my arms up over his neck. Because I was having a hard time walking, I leaned into him as he half dragged me to the bathroom. I was giggling the whole way and it felt good to laugh; it felt even better to hear Jeff laughing along with me. After I used the bathroom, Jeff helped me up to wash my hands. I was so loopy by then from the medicine that I couldn't stop laughing. My focus went to the water and I watched my hands move in slow motion as I told Jeff I was swimming and couldn't leave the sink. We laughed and laughed as he finally pulled me out of the bathroom and got me settled back in bed. Little did I know, he was taking a video of me playing in the water. It was cute to see Jeff getting such a kick out of my silliness, even in my loopy state.

Things had been so hard on him and it was nice to see Jeff laughing along with my craziness and I was grateful I had this medicine to lift me out of the darkness. Was this the way the rest of my life would be? I guess I could get through it as long as I had Jeff by my side. I relied on him so much and although it made me feel bad, he always made me feel like helping me was no big deal at all. His love was all I needed.

After about an hour, the giggles wore off and the medicine slowly melted away. Then I was drowsy and ready for bed. As Jeff said our nightly prayer, I silently pleaded with God to help me find anything to get better. I didn't care what it was but I begged Him to guide me to something that could heal me on a deeper level.

CHAPTER 20

SURRENDER

"Maybe it's time to call my buddy Jared again and see what his wife Elle did to heal her body," said Jeff. "Remember, he was telling me she went and did some kind of treatment and it really helped her?"

My husband was giving me that concerned look—the one that said he could tell that I wasn't at the end of my tether . . . I was at the end of the last, fragmented string to that tether.

"Just give me her number," I said wearily. "I want to hear her story directly from her. Especially as she was sicker than me and you said now she's feeling great and isn't sick anymore. That's hard to believe, but I remember . . . she was bedridden." I glanced from the bed up into my husband's eyes. "Get me her number. I am desperate." There was no please or smile followed by my words, just pure irritation that I was having to seek yet another treatment.

I didn't know Elle well, but I knew she had been sick for years lying in bed. By all accounts, she had been even worse off than I was. I had only heard a little here and there from Jeff, but he wasn't always the best at getting details from his friend about his wife's health.

The next evening after Jeff was done with work, I shuffled into Jeff's chilly office, the only quiet place in the house where no one would hear the conversation I was about to have. His office was tucked off of our bedroom with shiplap walls and a cluttered desk. I glanced out the window to see another cold, dreary day. I was longing for spring and was counting down the days until January would finally be over. Jeff was hanging out with the kids while I made the call in privacy since I wasn't sure how the conversation would go. I called Elle and was greeted by the sweetest, most tender voice on the other end of the line, so I started in. "Elle, it's Brita, Jeff's wife; he gave me your number. Can you please tell me your story? I would love to hear what you've done to heal your body." There was no point in wasting time, I wanted to get straight to the point and hear her story to see if this could help me as well.

As her story unfolded, I found myself sitting in Jeff's uncomfortable office chair, my jaw gaping open. I wasn't sure what to expect from her, but I admit, it sounded pretty weird! She had gone out of the country and tried ayahuasca at a healing retreat center in Costa Rica. I listened intently as she told me how she went from bedridden to slowly getting off all of her meds and getting pain-free. I couldn't believe it when she also told me her depression was gone and she was living a happy, fulfilled life. It was even more amazing that she had been feeling this good for three years now. The thought of feeling good for three whole years really made me very interested to give this a try, even though I was a little hesitant.

Can this really be true?

"That is amazing, Elle, it's hard to believe, I'm a little confused. How does plant medicine work?" I posed the question, my mind flooding with so much new information I was having a hard time processing it all.

"You can read more about it, but it basically puts your ego aside and your mind goes to work healing things you may not even be aware of with the use of psilocybin," Elle continued.

She was explaining everything so patiently, but I had never heard of this before and grasping the concept took a little more explaining. "Okay, so are you able to remember anything after you wake up?"

"You aren't asleep," Elle clarified. "You remember everything you experience, so you don't need to worry about being drugged or anything. The medicine shows you what you need to see. For example, I went into medicine with the intention to heal my body and I was shown and felt some intense experiences that helped me heal. It doesn't always make sense at the time, but before, during and after the medicine, I have processed the pain, anger and frustration that I had been suppressing."

"Interesting . . ." I laughed nervously. Even though I didn't know Elle well, she was being so kind as I tried to wrap my head around this. "So I still don't know exactly how it works, but I will remember what I go through?"

"Yes, you will remember it all," Elle assured me.

I was a little weirded out, but the fact that Elle's depression was gone was convincing enough for me to at least give it a try. I wasn't sure how to move forward but said, "Wow, this is really interesting. How would I go about scheduling an appointment?"

But there was more. Elle's journey hadn't stopped there. She let me know she had trained to become a Shaman and could guide me through a plant medicine ceremony herself.

I thanked her for sharing so openly and vulnerably with me, my eyes still wide as I just sat there, my head cocked to the side. I was skeptical. I was skeptical. Oh yes, I was skeptical . . . but suddenly I figured that if *she* could get better, then maybe I could, too. At this point, I didn't have anything to lose.

I wasn't sure exactly what I was getting myself into, but I felt very strongly that this was the next step for me and I put my trust in Elle as I planned for an upcoming session.

"I think I would like to give this a try," I said hesitantly. "Can you explain what I'll be doing?"

"You'll be taking a substance called psilocybin, or mushrooms. It's a psychedelic, so it will help you get to your subconscious to safely work through repressed emotions and experiences. What's most important is for you to prepare an intention for the session—what you most highly desire to receive by doing this. I'll explain cutting out certain foods and eating clean to prepare your body for your best experience."

I took that in as she explained she was booked up for a bit and the soonest she could get me in was March. So, I had three months to pray and prepare. She also talked to me about the long questionnaire I would need to fill out to make sure it would be safe for me to participate in a session.

"I think I can make that work," I said, only a little disappointed to have to wait. "Let me know the date and double check with Jeff and I will get back to you." I paused, slightly overwhelmed with emotion. "Thank you, Elle, for taking the time to talk to me about this. I have been praying to know what to do next and I'm shocked that this is it! I really appreciate you sharing your story with me. It's fascinating to hear how well you are doing."

We ended the call shortly after and I sat in silence for a few minutes to gather my thoughts.

To say I was scared was the understatement of the year. Growing up a good Christian girl who followed almost every rule, agreeing to do plant medicine felt like I was doing something *wrong*. My conditioning told me that I was going against everything I had learned! Here I was, trying something that I knew little about, but I felt like I couldn't tell anyone what I was doing. Except for Jeff, of course; I couldn't wait to tell him about my conversation with Elle. But I wouldn't tell anyone else what I was up to. I felt I had to be very secretive for my sake and for Elle, since not everyone was open to plant medicine.

Heck, I wasn't even open to plant medicine until ten minutes ago! I don't even know what a Shaman is.

I found Jeff shortly after my conversation with Elle. My husband could see the amusement on my face, including my awkward smile and raised eyebrows. He smiled back at me, anxious to hear what Elle had to say. "How did it go?" Jeff asked.

"Well, it's weird. But I want to do it," I said as we both laughed.

I recalled the conversation I had with Elle, trying to explain everything as well as I could remember. Jeff sat silently nodding his head and only interjecting with "interesting" here and there.

"Honestly, Jeff, I feel weird committing to this, but she has an opening in March and I feel very strongly I should do this. There is a part of me that feels like I'm doing something bad, but the other part of me is screaming at me to go for it."

Jeff wrapped me up in a hug, saying, "You've always been guided to the next steps and this feels like a good choice to me. I love you so much and hope this helps you."

I felt a rush of warmth. Once again, I was grateful for Jeff's love and support, the one person I could talk to about anything. He was ready for me to feel better and if this is what it took, then he was all in.

After lots of internet searching and reading, I found out that Shamanism was a spiritual practice that involves a healer interacting with what they believe to be a spirit world, through altered states of consciousness.

To be honest, it sounded a bit wacky to me. *Still, what do I have to lose?* That was a phrase I was saying way too much. I beat my head against a door in my mind. After all, I had tried everything else! I had exhausted the western medicine world of multiple prescriptions and side-effects, invasive surgeries and long years of therapy. Then I'd moved to natural supplements and oils, fasting, infrared saunas and hyperbaric chambers. So far, everything I heard about, I gave it a try. I was ready to take the next chance here.

Although many of my treatments helped to some extent, everything was temporary. I couldn't find one treatment that could help me *stay better*. We decided not to tell any of our family or friends that I was going to try plant medicine. Jeff and I weren't interested in their opinions since they really didn't know how much I was suffering. And no matter what anyone else said, I was doing it anyway.

So I patiently, or rather, impatiently waited for March as my body ached and my mind spiraled. For the first time in a very long while, however, I felt a sense of hope. I sat down at my computer to fill out the long questionnaire to take part in the plant medicine session where I took full responsibility for any adverse reactions I might have, even death. I shuddered as I read that line, but was determined to do anything if it meant my life would be better than it was. I couldn't live like I was any longer.

As I was anxious for March to come, I had a close friend, Angie, who opened up to me about her experience with Kanna, another psychedelic drug that she had used to begin to heal from her past. I was shocked when she told me about this, since I had known her for about eighteen years and never would have guessed she was going down this road. She was a petite, blonde-haired, beautiful soul and I was grateful she would open up to me about her experience. She was studying to get her master's as a therapist and offered to guide me through a psychedelic experience as early as February. Breathlessly, I realized that our connection was not a coincidence. I nervously set a date to work with her one on one and see what would come up during the session.

Like Elle, Angie guided me to set intentions for the session. I chose my intention quickly: *to heal my heart and body.* I was dealing with so many health issues, it finally seemed fitting—made actual, rational and logical sense to me now—to see if there was a root cause that I hadn't been able to heal completely and therefore was the reason for my constant relapses of agony and sickness.

"Plant medicine is a process," Angie explained gently to my questioning. "You have to process things before the session, during it and then after. It's a lot of work." Her voice now contained a warning: "This is not an easy, relaxing healing modality, Brita."

"Okay," I said, but I had no idea what to expect.

Angie also let me know she had trained as a Shaman and would be guiding me through this not only as a studying therapist, but also as a religious ceremony. I wasn't sure what that meant, but after Elle and now Angie and my desperation, I was open to anything.

Because of the nature of the Kanna, I was to go spend the night with Angie to have a session with her. Leading up to that evening, I was very nervous to go. I had a weird feeling that kept making me question if I was doing the right thing. I knew that sometimes we have to experience the death of something old in order to create the birth of something new. If I could die off an old part of me to create a life I loved and could finally embrace fully, I was ready. Still anxious, but ready.

I entered Angie's beautiful, bright home, where she gave me a warm and loving hug as her yellow Lab bounded up to me wagging his tail. I pet her friendly dog as I took my shoes off and unloaded my pillow and bag in her entry. Angie told me her kids were gone and we were the only ones here. Then she guided me to her comfy couch in her front room where I snuggled up with the soft blanket I had brought from home. Even though I trusted her, I was still very nervous. I trembled a little as I handed over cash to pay for the session and waited for things to begin.

We talked for a few minutes and my fears and nervousness melted away as I could feel her love for me. I breathed out, not realizing I had been holding my breath. *I am in the best place for more healing.* Angie lowered the blinds and turned the lights down low, lighting a few candles to create a more calming space. She turned on some beautiful "yoga" music that filled me with comfort, since music had always meant so much to me.

Angie sat close and said, "Remember, this is a sacred medicine. It is only something you should do in the right setting, with someone who is experienced and I will be here with you the whole time to support you."

Angie handed me the pill to swallow and I closed my eyes as I held it in my hand for a moment. Silently, I prayed: *Dear Father, please guide me during this session that I will be safe and protected. Please help me to see what I need to see and know what I need to know so that I can heal my body. Thank you for guiding me here. Please help me feel Your peace and be with me.* I swallowed the pill and waited to see what would happen.

As I ingested my first dose of psychedelics, I had no idea what to expect. I was grateful that I was in a one-on-one session with a trained professional and a friend by my side, guiding me through it. At first, I started to feel weird and somehow . . . lighter. Angie turned the volume up on the nice, relaxing music to help my ego relax, dropping me into a different level of consciousness.

At first, I spoke up, requesting she write down what I was saying as I was lying down in the dimly lit room. I asked her to write letters to my children and Jeff, because the love I felt for them was even more intense in this state.

Slowly, I got deeper and deeper into the medicine. Then, Angie's big yellow dog came and stood by me and the hair on my neck stood up. My body tensed up, not wanting the dog to touch me. He came up, uninvited and rubbed his nose on my knee and I flinched, moving my knee away. An overpowering feeling of fear hit me and I blurted, "Angie, your dog is freaking me out; can you put him away, please?"

Angie called her dog to lay down in his bed, but I still felt paranoid as I kept eyeing the dog. As an animal lover, it didn't make sense to me that I was suddenly scared of her dog. I eyed the creature laying in the bed a few feet in front of me and all I wanted was for him to get out of the house, far away from me. I didn't like the way he was looking at me. I tried to ignore him, but for some reason he was making my body stay tense and ready to run if I needed to.

My mind finally wandered from the dog, but abruptly focused on the male voice singing through the speaker. His voice penetrated my body and my fear became even more exaggerated. "I'm scared," I admitted, my voice getting quiet and high-pitched more like a child. I felt thirsty all of a sudden and asked Angie to hand me my water bottle, then I demanded, "Turn off that music, he's scaring me."

"I can see that you are scared, Brita," Angie said gently, "and I can turn off the music if you want me to, but what is scaring you?"

"His voice!" I cried louder, almost shouting. "His voice is scaring me!"

Just then I felt a gentle touch as Angie held my hand. She said softly, "You are safe; it's only you and me here. I can turn the music off so you can feel better . . . *or* you can discover why this music is making you feel this way. The man singing is nice and is singing to beautiful music. Do you want to keep going to see why you are afraid?"

I took a couple deep breaths and found curiosity rising within me. I felt like I did want to discover more of what was making me so scared. I took a couple deep breaths, remembering I was safe and in good hands.

"Keep the music on," I said, now determined. It was as if I declared I was officially ready. All of a sudden, waves of fear, anger, disgust, terror, shame and guilt all started moving through me. I knew I wasn't reliving an experience, but I felt like I certainly was reliving emotions of something that had happened . . . something long, long ago.

Suddenly, I started sobbing harder than I had ever cried in my life.

"Are you okay?" Angie asked.

"No, I'm not okay. HE HURT ME!" I cried so hard that my face hurt and my body was so stiff as the tears cascaded down my cheeks.

"Who hurt you?" she guided me.

I said his name. The name of the man who sexually abused me at three years old.

It was as if my body was telling me a scary story that I didn't want to hear. The man who was a close friend of our family. The man who was supposed to be safe and was not. The man I had heard my dad talk about, what a good guy he was. I gasped as I cried out in the realization that this was a memory so deeply hidden that I could only find it in this setting, under these circumstances, with Angie as my guide.

I cried more and spoke all the unspoken that I had held onto for years. I talked to Angie for quite some time, processing through these excruciating emotions that felt so heavy in my brittle body.

As the emotions were released and the terror and tension in my body began to subside, little by little, I was amazed. The intention I came into this session with was to heal. This memory, this deep, deep betrayal was the last thing I ever expected to come up. It was heart-wrenching for me to discover this about this man, about the truth of my childhood and his taking of my innocence. And the realization that he had taken my power all the way back then—not all of it, but the power over my body? Yes.

The weird thing I discovered about being on the psychedelic was that even though I was scared and feeling so many emotions, I also felt *safe* to discover and talk about it all. I could process deep, high and low and heavy emotions while knowing my physical and mental safety were already contained for me. It took me about six hours in that session, talking and working through this traumatic event and a whole lot of other stuff that came up in which several of the puzzle pieces of my life began to come together.

Before I fell asleep, I grabbed the notebook I had brought with me and began writing. Out poured everything that was on my mind. I felt like I was writing for hours but eventually I was able to drift off to sleep and woke up groggily the next morning. As I glanced at the notebook I had written in, I laughed to myself as I didn't see many words, but instead there were mainly scribbles.

I distinctly remembered writing so many words the night before, but when I looked at the paper, it looked like a young child had sat doodling nonsense all over the page. I was surprised when I also noticed the number three circled a few times on the page.

It dawned on me that the scared little girl from my past was coming out on paper. I shivered as chills ran down my spine and arms. After carefully setting down my notebook, I headed upstairs to where Angie had a nice breakfast ready for me. I was so nauseated, I could hardly eat. I didn't know if I was sick from the medicine, or the news I uncovered. It was probably a mixture of both.

My friend and I talked about what had been discovered in the medicine. Now back to my normal state of mind, everything made so much sense! I always had a question in the back of my mind, wondering if I had ever been sexually abused, but because I had no memories of it in my waking state, I always shrugged it off.

Now I knew what had happened to me. I knew why I had shoved those memories down into the far reaches of my consciousness to survive. This was something I didn't want to remember because it was so awful, but now I was anxious to continue healing.

When Jeff came to pick me up, he gathered me into his arms with a warm and loving hug. I was so grateful to have him there to support me.

Because Jeff knew Angie well, he stayed to visit before we left to go back home. Angie started the conversation by saying, "Jeff, what do you think about Brita doing this?"

Jeff looked at me lovingly, then looked back at Angie. "I am so proud of her."

I smiled at Jeff as he was there for me once again, with no judgment. It felt so good to hear that he was proud of me. I wondered how he would react when I told him about the session. We said our goodbyes to Angie, giving her hugs and thanking her for all she had done for me. Jeff gathered my blanket and pillow. As we walked outside, he put them in the car and then opened the door for me to sink in. I was exhausted.

"How did it go?" Jeff asked anxiously. "Was it how you thought it would be?"

He was talking fast, which was unusual for him and I could tell he was hoping this had helped. My words came out a lot slower. "Well, it was very weird, but cool and very different than I thought it would be. I had quite an intense experience that I was not expecting." I paused as I took a long drink of my water. I felt parched. I told him what happened with Angie's dog and how the music had triggered something buried deep within me. I paused again and started crying.

He glanced at me with a concerned look, his head tilting to the side, "Are you okay?" he gently spoke.

"Yes and no. It's hard to explain, but I had so many yucky emotions flood my body. That's when I knew I had been sexually abused when I was little." Saying this out loud made the tears flow again. I sat and cried silently as Jeff reached over and held my hand, not saying anything but just being there for me. His thumb glided softly over my skin as I continued to cry for a few more minutes trying to compose myself.

When I was able to catch my breath again, I cried out, "I'm so angry! What kind of man does that to a little girl? Just what kind of man?" I beat my hands upon my knees. "And it's so weird because I don't have any memories of it. The only thing I remember about him is one evening before dinner, he wiped cologne on my nose and it ruined dinner for me. Don't ask me how I can remember that since I was only three years old. But it was very clear in the medicine that he hurt me—that he hurt me so badly. I felt every feeling, Jeff. Most of the session was processing that experience. It was very intense."

My husband could see how exhausted I was emotionally and physically. He didn't ask any questions and just said, "I'm so sorry," as he continued to rub my hand as we drove back home.

I wasn't in the mood to talk more right then. I needed a long nap before I could talk more. We had told our kids that I was getting a treatment, which was very normal for me, so they weren't surprised when I walked in the house exhausted and needed to lie down. I got hugs from the kids and passed out quickly. But the processing was not over.

CHAPTER 21

RISE FROM THE ASHES

The days following that first session with Angie were full of harsh, honest questions.

Wow, was that real?

Did he really hurt me in that way?

It was hard to believe, yet I certainly didn't have any reason to make it up, especially since he was trusted by my family. My parents thought he was a nice guy. They had no reason to expect anything was going on.

I started doubting my experience. How could something so awful happen to me and I couldn't remember it at all? There were many questions that kept flooding my mind each day. Slowly, I was learning that I had to feel it all deeply in order to heal and it was not easy. I felt like I was emotional all the time.

Angie was right. I continued to process and process long and hard after my experience. The truth that kept percolating through was that this abuse indeed had happened and it had spiraled much of my life out of control. I was shocked and disgusted while I tried to continue to understand what had been unearthed.

March came quickly and I found myself in Elle's home, nervous for my second plant medicine experience. This time, I would be ingesting a tea made from mushrooms, or psilocybin, instead of a pill. Also, instead of a one-on-one session, I would be in a group with two other people. I was very nervous to do a session with others, feeling a little self-conscious.

Elle made me feel comfortable right away as she gave me a warm hug as I stepped into her home. Walking past the front room, Elle introduced me to one of her helpers named Sara, who was tall and had long blonde hair. She gave me a welcoming smile and greeted me in a friendly way. Next, I met the other two people who were doing the session with me. They were husband and wife and were relatives of Elle.

Elle guided us all downstairs to her basement, past the bathroom, then into a large room where we would be doing the session. The basement was dimly lit and Elle showed us where we could put our blankets and pillows on the floor right by each other along the back wall of the room. I chose the farthest spot from the stairs and the wife was in the middle, the husband farthest from me. We were all shifting and looking around, trying to figure out what to do next.

Elle called each of us upstairs one at a time to talk with her and Sara to go over our intentions. When it was my turn, I sat down on a comfy armchair facing the two women.

"Remind me what your intention is?" Elle asked.

"To heal my body," I said as tears welled up in my eyes.

Elle leaned over and held my hand. "It's okay, love. We are here for you and I know you will find the answers you are seeking. Just ask the medicine what you need to see and know and you will be guided right where you need to be. We will be right there if you need anything."

During this ceremony that Elle performed, we had to take a vow of silence, which was very different from my first session where I talked everything through with Angie. Since I was very comforted by talking with Angie through my first session, I was worried that it would be difficult to process emotions while being silent. I said a silent prayer. *God, I know You have guided me here, but I don't know what to expect. Please calm my heart and help me to continue to heal.* I had no idea what to expect and so starting out, I was already a little weirded out by the whole thing. Still, it was important to me to go through with it.

As I sat silently in the dark basement focusing on my intention, I started to relax and was ready to get going.

Elle and Sara came downstairs and started the ceremony. Elle said, "You may notice the buckets at the end of your blankets. They are there just in case you feel like you need to throw up. Part of the plant medicine experience may be purging. That can come in many forms like vomiting, burping, laughing, pooping . . ." She giggled then continued, "It's pretty rare to vomit with this medicine, but anything can happen. Did you all see the bathroom right at the bottom of the stairs?"

We all nodded that we had. I had already used the restroom three times, thanks to my nervous bladder.

Elle continued, "You might feel a little unsteady once you take the medicine, so if you need any help, just raise your hand and we will come help you out. We are here to support you so don't hesitate to raise your hand if you need anything."

Elle called us up one by one to take the medicine. The mushrooms were mixed with orange juice, but *ugh,* it did not taste good and was hard to swallow. Still, after gagging a little, I laid on the carpet with my blanket and a pillow. I focused on my breathing and closed my eyes.

It didn't take long for the medicine to kick in and soon, I felt like I was in a dreamlike state. Intense emotions came at me, like waves were hitting me in the face without time to catch my breath. Sadness rolled through me first. I sobbed for what felt like quite a long time. Sara came and sat by me, placing her hand on my back as my shoulders heaved. It felt nice to have someone by me while I cried.

I had the realization that in my waking state for my whole life and even in the month since my first experience, I had repressed a lot of anger, sadness and fear. Somehow I had cut myself off from parts of me. I had never allowed myself to feel anything quite like this. For decade upon decade, I stuffed my emotions and pain down deep inside myself and suffered in silence.

The plant medicine put my ego to sleep and slapped me in the face with the strongest emotions I had ever felt. The next waves that splashed into me were rage and disgust. Sara came back by me and I gave her a death glare, not wanting her to touch me this time. She sensed my anger and didn't touch me, but sat close in case I needed her.

As my feelings rose with such intensity, so did my nausea. I puked my guts out in the bucket near my feet. I remembered that purging, however, can be a vital part of any plant ceremony session and apparently, this was what my body needed. I could tell because I was purging like crazy.

About halfway through the ceremony, the medicine started to wear off and we were given the opportunity to take a second dose. Even though the original dose was already kicking my butt and I could have been satisfied with what I was already experiencing, I was determined to do as much healing as I could.

Standing up, I accepted another dose and was instantly nauseated. I stepped unsteadily to my little bed on the floor and immediately started puking up in my bucket again. I had never puked so much in my life and yet I knew it: I was releasing so much more than the physical element of the mushrooms and juice.

While I was vomiting, I could feel all eyes on me, but I wasn't able to get my head out of the bucket long enough to see what the others' expressions were. I was too busy to react.

Then the most incredible thing happened. With my head in the bucket, a powerful phrase shouted inside my head:

You don't need medicine to heal! You don't need medicine to heal!

That powerful truth rushed through me. It was suddenly so clear to me that *this* medicine—so different from the pharmaceuticals that had often completely enshrouded my life—was reminding me of *my* power, reminding me that I could reach within myself to heal. *I* was my medicine.

I was overcome with joy at this realization. It was so refreshing! I felt empowered. It was crazy, here with my head in the bucket and yet I had never been so happy to be throwing up. I knew without one shadow of a doubt that I was getting out all the negativity, all the pain, all the things I was never able to say or yell or cry—and now all of it combined together was coming out of my mouth. It was so symbolic to my healing.

Along with this sense of surety, I realized it was time to find my voice and be my true, authentic self—without covering up or pretending that everything was okay when it wasn't, or being hurt when others didn't accept my expressed pain or fears. I had never experienced such a powerful urge to fight through it all. I felt that fire rise up in me. I knew I was healing and I had never been prouder of myself for showing up and facing whatever was to come.

After I had gotten the second dose completely out of my system, Elle came to make sure I was okay. I took a few deep breaths and said with confidence, "Yes, I can do this."

Elle then offered me a third dose and to my amazement and awe, I discovered my body was ready for it this time. Even though I truly knew I had the power in me to heal now, I knew I needed this to get through my ego. This was the most important work for me to do through the plant medicine while I had this opportunity. Without hesitation, I drank the liquid and laid in the bed again.

Empowered with my new knowledge, something within me began to shift. This time as I was lying there, my mind started to go into the dreamlike state again. Countless doctors had been trying to fix what they could see for so many years, but that wasn't the only part that needed fixing. It was only in this medicine that I could find the broken parts that needed to be healed. A new awareness developed.

Before this dose, every time I had to use the bathroom or get up at all, I would raise my hand and Sara or Elle would hold onto me so I didn't fall down when I walked. I felt like I had to rely on someone to help me since the medicine was pretty intense. I happened to look over at the woman in the session with me. She got up on her own and walked to the bathroom on her own! A thrill of deepest fire shot through me. Seeing her do that gave me the courage to stand on my own—physically and emotionally. When it was time for me to get up, I leaned on the wall to brace myself, then I marched to the bathroom without any help.

I was making progress. I was so damn proud of it!

Then I laid back down, equally committed to the final part of my experience. This session was full of processing the sexual assault and also a lot of feelings I had of not being seen and heard. I had heard that autoimmune diseases were often caused by feelings of powerlessness, to protect ourselves from some energy or enemy.

That idea rang so true for me and I allowed myself to be curious and explore it. Could my autoimmune diseases have been caused by this trauma? Had my body been reacting to feeling unsafe and unprotected? It made sense.

A short time after processing and accepting this new knowledge, some new realizations and emotions came up. Flashes of other memories and strong emotions welled up inside of me and I allowed myself to experience grief from my miscarriage. It was extraordinary and I felt a growing closeness to that love that I had carried within me, the love that I was never able to hold in my hands and lost before giving a name. It was such a tender experience once I allowed the sharp anguish I had shoved down in my past to wash over me, so I could heal it.

That was not a fun or relaxing session. It was intense and painful, but in the midst of it, I could feel, little by little, that I was healing the innermost parts of me.

After what seemed like a week and not just a few hours, I began coming out of the session. As the medicine worked its way out of our bodies, the group of us gathered in Elle's dining room to enjoy some fruit, soup and bread while we talked about our experiences. I could only eat a little. We laughed as Elle and her helpers commented on all the puking I did, which was apparently so out of the ordinary. My cheeks burned a little as they declared they were proud when I got up and walked on my own to the bathroom. I was delighted to be in their company as I continued to deeply process the experience and witness other healing that took place too.

Once again, my husband picked me up. I was grateful and thankful to see Jeff and on the way home, I told him everything that went on in my session. I cried and laughed as I told him how I processed the childhood trauma again, more deeply this time. I shared the acceptance and the empowerment. With several honest tears, I shared how I grieved for the pregnancy I lost. The entire time, my amazing husband held my hand. Though he didn't tear up along with me, I could feel the tenderness and grief coming through in his comforting words. The whole ride, he simply showered me with his love and I was finally able to receive it. I couldn't believe how lucky I was to have him in my life.

Braver now as weeks passed, I decided to continue on my path of healing by committing to three more plant medicine ceremonies: two more with Angie and the Kanna and one more session with Elle and the psilocybin.

Each experience was so different and amazing, so healing and beautiful. Little by little, I was getting more vital energy in my body. To my amazement and delight, after three sessions, I found that my depression was gone. I was shocked since I had been battling my mind for *so long*. Feeling happy and mentally stable was such a blessing.

I was honestly not expecting these sessions to heal my depression, as deep inside I wasn't sure it would ever go away. To be free of the heavy shackles of depression made me feel like my life was full of promise again.

After one of these sessions, I had spoken to Jeff and told him that I would never be able to forgive the man who abused me. What he had done was too awful and sickening. I felt completely justified in not forgiving him and didn't think it was a necessary part of healing.

Sure, growing up a Christian, I learned that forgiveness was important, but I couldn't see how it was going to be that way for me. I was too hurt. I felt that this man was the root cause of most of my health issues, depression and all the suffering I had been experiencing–for decades. He didn't deserve to be forgiven! I knew God would love me even if I couldn't forgive and I had no intention of doing so.

After I finished my five sessions, I processed and healed so much each time. I gave myself permission to continue to feel my emotions in my everyday life. This was new for me. I prayed that I would be guided to continue to heal my heart and my body. If I was sad, I honored that feeling and I sat and cried. For the first time in my life, I didn't shove it down. I no longer ignored the feelings. My heart began to soften toward myself. All the feelings of hate that I had toward myself and my body were slowly melting away.

I was still in the same body with the same mind, but it was amazing—I could finally look in the mirror and like who I saw. I was able to forgive myself for not being the wife and mother I had planned to be. I forgave myself for being so hard on myself when I had to stay in bed to rest instead of being out with my family. I forgave myself for hiding under my covers instead of dealing with the pain of what was really going on.

I thanked myself for never giving up and being able to keep getting up to fight. I could look into my own eyes and smile and say, "Brita, I love you. Thank you for showing up today." I allowed myself to rest when I needed and let go of all the expectations I had of myself. I gave myself patience and kindness, something I hadn't done for myself in a really long time. I was free. I freed myself from the darkness and I promised myself to always take care of me first, which was no longer hard for me to do.

As I continued to love myself, my heart slowly began to soften. One day, as I was praying, I was surprised at what came out.

"Dear Father, I have been so angry and so disgusted at the man who hurt me to my core. Right now I feel like he took everything from me and I hate him because of it. It is so clear to me that all of my pain is linked to this trauma that he put me through and I'm so, so angry. I haven't wanted to forgive him because I felt like it would mean it didn't happen, that he was off the hook. And I wanted him to suffer.

"I wanted him to feel the pain I felt over and over again, like I somehow had the power to do that through my own suffering. I have realized that I have no power over him, but he has had power over me. I don't want him to have any power over me anymore."

I took a deep breath, then let it out slowly. "So . . . I want to forgive him. Through You, Father and only You, I choose to forgive him. Please help him find healing. I don't want to carry this pain around with me anymore. I don't want to hold onto hate anymore. Please take this hate away and replace it with Your love. I know that I need Your help to forgive him; please be with me."

As I continued, I felt a new truth and fire rising up within me. This time it wasn't a spark, it wasn't just a flame, it was a roaring fire of truth.

"I am done being the victim. I am finished giving away any of my power. Instead, I want to carry this around with me as armor, to catch others on fire with the light in my soul instead of it dragging me down. I give this to You and I will tell my story as I continue to heal. I will help others own their story and their voice because I know how hard it is. Thank You, Father, for Your grace and strength you have given me when I didn't have any for myself. I love You."

CHAPTER 22

BEAUTIFUL BROKEN

The alarm clock went off and I slowly rolled over to turn it off. Seven already? I quietly got out of bed, since Jeff was still sleeping and listened to see if the kids were up for school. One by one, my kids came downstairs to greet me before they headed off for their day. Jeff joined us in the living room shortly after, in time for us both to give our kids loving hugs before they headed out to school. When the house was quiet, Jeff and I sat on the couch for a few minutes talking about the day ahead of us. Jeff was heading to the gym for a workout. I was going for a walk at the park, then we would come home and start working for the day where we both worked from home.

The walk at the park was a nice start to my day and I enjoy the beautiful trees all around the park and I was so happy to be walking in the fall air before the leaves had fallen. There was something about school starting back up and the cool mornings that energized me. I reflected on the last several years where I wasn't able to enjoy mornings like this and tears came to my eyes in gratitude, being so thankful to have the energy to be walking around the park. I may not have been going fast, but I was moving this amazing body that was still there to hold me up.

It was hard to believe how much things had changed in my mind and body. I laughed to myself, feeling such deep happiness—no longer covered in a film of depression, no longer pushing through the sludge of brain fog. My mind felt light and capable, a feeling I had missed for way too long. I was surprised once again to feel better after my walk was over, instead of drained and tired, no longer feeling the heaviness of the trauma I had experienced and replacing it with the lightness of forgiveness for myself and others. I had been beating myself up for years for the ways I wasn't showing up for my kids and husband. But I tried not to focus on that and reminded myself that I was doing my best and that was all I could do. Even in my toughest moments, I just did the best I could. Accepting myself just as I was, it was a good feeling I had longed to feel.

The drive home from the park was short. I took a quick shower and sat down at my desk to look at my planner and what was ahead of me for the day.

First, I had to work for a while, for the livestock company, Brazzen, that I worked for. I needed to call some of our customers, create some brochures and flyers and make some updates on the company website and other tasks that were on my to-do list. I continued looking at my planner where a busy day was ahead of me. After school, Avery had karate, Carter had football and soccer practice, Taylor had horse lessons and Callen needed to do some driving since he had just gotten his driving permit. Landan was now graduated from high school, working and taking care of herself, which was a weird transition for me. But, I was excited for the day, knowing I would have the energy to take everyone where they needed to go.

It was such a change from even a year ago, where I was still spending so much time in my bed. The workday went by fast and before I knew it, four of the kids were home (Landan was still at work) where we gathered to talk about each of their days. This was my favorite part of the day, having them home from school and chatting about anything that went on. Everyone got ready for their activities, drop-offs and pickups happened and dinner was made as we all sat together to eat a quick meal before the last few activities we had to get to.

As we were eating dinner, I looked around the happy faces at the dinner table and I couldn't believe how happy we all were. It almost didn't feel real to be here. There were so many struggles for so long and so many days where my family brought me dinner in my bed because I didn't have the energy to join them at the table. In those moments, I never imagined I would feel this good again.

Each of my children were growing up to be such kind, compassionate, incredible children who were patient and independent. Through all the struggles, they had become amazing people that I loved. I was so grateful to be a part of their lives, that I was still here enjoying my time with them, out of bed and with them. I soaked in all the laughter and chatter with my family, enjoying each of my kids with how different they were from each other, each unique and wonderful in their own ways. I was so proud to call them mine.

Before I knew it, everyone was in bed and Jeff and I sat talking about our day. I leaned into Jeff's arms as we talked and felt so safe and blessed.

This man who had been by my side through so much adversity had so many burdens placed on him and he was still such a loving man who I adored. We laughed and talked about our day, dreaming about our future where Jeff was encouraging me to finish my book to share my story with others.

I felt free. A body that was healing, my depression was gone, it was such an adjustment to the life I had gotten used to in the past. My prayers to end the night were full of gratitude and I sobbed as I thanked God for getting me here and for helping me get through each hard day and find the strength to continue on, when I wasn't sure I would be able to. I felt so incredibly blessed to be living such a beautiful life that I loved.

CHAPTER 23

DISCOVER THE BEAUTY
IN BEING BROKEN

When I say broken, I mean broken down to my core to be rebuilt into a version of myself that wouldn't have existed without the struggles. I wish I could have seen more of the beauty along the way but I was too busy being mad about everything I was lacking, focused on everything I couldn't do. My hope is that I can help people like me to see the beauty in their life even if it's different than they wanted. I don't know if anyone could have reached me or helped me when I was in the midst of my biggest storms. But I will try my best to keep throwing out rafts so if even one person can be saved then I will keep sharing my story to let people know that they aren't alone—to build a supportive and kind community where they can feel safe.

The thing is, in the midst of my sadness and suffering, I didn't see the beauty surrounding me. But as I have transformed and healed parts of me, now I can see the beauty in all the brokenness. Believe me, when I was going through it I didn't see it. Instead, I beat myself up and told myself I wasn't good enough because I could only lie in bed. Sometimes, I was mean, sad and felt like I wasn't even good enough to breathe. But that's the beauty of it. We don't have to DO anything to be enough. We can just be. We are enough just as we are. No matter if we are sick or healthy, depressed or mentally stable. We may be different but we are beautiful people on our own path.

There are many things that I have realized in my journey that I'd love to share in a powerful list here. I have come up with the following strategies that might help someone else along their way as these have helped me. I hope you can also find the beauty in being broken and have the courage to be broken with me.

1. CHOOSE TO BE GRATEFUL

I used to cringe every time someone would tell me to be more grateful. *Ugh.* My mind would immediately go to "They don't get what I'm going through at all. Don't they know that I'm grateful for what I have and I'm still struggling?" But as I've looked back on my journey, being grateful is such an important focus, especially for chronically ill people. I've always felt so blessed to have an amazing husband and kids by my side during the ups and the downs. My parents and siblings have been such a huge support to me. I'm so grateful for them. I'm also very grateful to have such a comfy bed to relax in, since I've spent so much time in it.

Being grateful may not change your circumstances, but it puts the focus on all the good in your life, which is important to acknowledge.

2. OUTWARD FOCUS

Before I got sick, I was a very motivated, caring person. I enjoyed serving those around me. Chronic illness was so hard to manage and I would find myself so self-consumed that it was hard to take care of anyone else. One thing I realized is there are so many ways that we can serve people right from our bed. I always did what I could for my kids and that felt good, but I found a handful of my friends just needed someone to text or talk to. Even when I wasn't feeling good, I could still send a nice message to my friends so they would know I was thinking of them. Sometimes I was too depressed to talk on the phone and I was honest with my friends about that. But it felt good to be there for others even if it was only in small ways and as I can do more, I do it. When I can't, I let the little things be big things because I took action.

Remember others and the world outside of your struggle and reach out.

3. BE TRUE TO YOURSELF

It's hard to set healthy boundaries with the ones you love. I have been lucky to have an amazing support system in place, but I know that not all people are so lucky. I have also had some very negative people in my life that I have learned to stay away from. This was especially true when I was dealing with depression and was barely holding myself together. When people around me would say things like "Things could always be worse" or "You need to choose to be happy," I would try to not take it personally. It was hard but very important to remind myself that those who said very insensitive things didn't always mean to hurt me. They often thought they were helping. So, instead of being hurt over and over again by the same people, I stopped hanging out with them. I'm sure they wondered why I wasn't coming around anymore, but for my own healing, I had to protect myself and take care of my own needs. I will be honest, before I got sick, I was terrible at setting boundaries. But when I got to the point where I only had so much energy to give, I found that it was more important to take care of my own needs than worrying about what anyone else needed from me.

Discover your boundaries and honor them.

4. BECOME A CREATOR

When I was in college, I took a lot of art classes for my major in Industrial Design (computer animation) and I loved them. As I graduated and transitioned into having a real job, I was grateful that I had chosen such a creative field to work in. Creating has always brought me so much joy. Whether it's designing a birthday invite for one of my kids or a flyer for work, I have found that I need to create to be happy. When I was drowning in depression so deep that I couldn't create anything, it really affected me. But even when I wasn't feeling good, I would drag myself to the piano and write a very sad song. It didn't always lift my mood, but it felt good to be creating something. Now when I create, I thank God that I am here and that my mind is able to be free to make new things. There was a time when it was almost impossible for me to create like I wanted to, but I can see the beauty in the sad songs I wrote. Music has always had a way of saying what I couldn't express through words.

Find your way to create.

5. ALLOW YOURSELF TO GRIEVE

If you suffer from a chronic illness like me, it's hard for others to understand that you need time to grieve the loss of your old self. There are many days when I look back at who I was in high school and college. I used to be fun and oozing with energy. Being happy was as easy as breathing. But once I got sick, I felt like I was trudging through thick mud most days.

It's okay to miss the things you could do and it's okay to be sad for the person you have lost. Grieve that loss and then move on and try to find happiness with who you have become. Allowing ourselves to be sad for what we lost is healthy, as long as we can pick up the pieces and find the new version of ourselves.

Give yourself time to process, but don't get stuck in your grief. Give it time and space but don't let it take you over.

6. THE BEAUTY OF EMOTIONS—FEEL IT ALL!

I have always been a very emotional person. I cry during commercials and get laughed at for doing so. For some reason, I grew up thinking that being an emotional person was something I had to hide and didn't feel that I could always express myself. When you bottle everything up, eventually you just explode. If you feel everything a little bit each day, it helps. Don't stick things in your pocket and ignore them, because eventually your pockets will be too full to carry it all. We need to keep our pockets light so we can run a little faster. Don't worry about what others think of you. Feel the good, bad and ugly emotions equally and be okay with how you need to process everything. Take care of yourself and don't worry about how other people think you need to be. You are the only one who truly knows what you need.

Be courageous and willing to feel your emotions and process them.

7. FORGIVENESS

This is one that has always been important to me, but I find it hard to forgive others when they hurt me so deeply. I have had many lessons in learning how to forgive. I rely on God to help me let go of the pain that I have been through on behalf of others. But one person that has been especially hard for me to forgive is myself. I was not the mom I dreamed I would be, my life stopped for so long and I was very disappointed in the life I was living. It has been so freeing to forgive myself for the things I can and can't control—for all the expectations I have had of myself.

Don't wait too long to forgive yourself and others, it sets you free in every way and helps you move forward happily.

8. DON'T GIVE UP ON YOURSELF

I have had many days when I was terribly hard on myself. When the negative talk would get bad, I tried to remind myself that I was doing my best and I needed to be nice and treat myself like a friend would. I didn't realize it at the time, but I was feeling like a victim through most of my health issues. I was angry that my life had turned out the way it was and I didn't like it. I felt sorry for myself and my kids. The day I was able to step out of that mindset was beautiful. Did it mean that my life was perfect? No. But I could see that I was in charge of my life and my thoughts. I didn't have to be miserable in my circumstances. There are some days it's really hard to not feel sorry for myself and all the things I wish were different, but when I step back and look at my life, I am so blessed. Something that has helped me is seeking direction through God. I pray a lot and it helps me find peace with where I'm at. I have been guided to try many treatments and different healing modalities and my best advice is to be open-minded and give things a try as long as your body and budget permit it. You might find something along the way that helps you, even though you were skeptical to try it.

Be open and willing to try new things. And never, never, never give up!

9. IT'S MORE FUN IF YOU LIKE IT!

Learning new things is a great way to distract yourself. After being a stay-at-home mom for years and being sick for years, I was ready to reenter the workforce when all my kids were in full time school. It was hard when I started working again, having to keep a schedule, learn new things and figure out how to work for a new boss. But I found that I loved learning and liked the challenge of problem-solving hard tasks. There might be a new hobby that you could learn to help pass the time. Be gentle with yourself as you try new things.

Bring wonder, discovery, learning and growth into your life. Discover what you truly love and enjoy.

10. GRASPING HOPE AGAIN

Even though I've had many hard days, I was determined to never give up completely. It has not been an easy road, but I am still walking slowly down it. During my athletic days, I always pushed myself to be the best. I trained hard and fought to be great at what I was doing. I've taken that same attitude as I've been forced to slow down. Even though I'm not out running every day, I still have to push myself in different ways. It's been important to engage my brain by setting new goals and finding activities that I *can* do. I might face more limitations in my future, but this I know about myself now: I will continue to get out of bed and accomplish what I can.

Each day, take a step. Find things to encourage you and set up realistic steps to move forward in while you celebrate something each day.

11. ACCEPTING YOUR LIFE

I'm not going to lie, it's been hard to accept my life. I never thought I would be a sick person stuck in bed. It never even crossed my mind when I was young. I never thought I would spend my 30s going to many doctor appointments, searching for answers and feeling shackled to my bed for most of it. It has taken me many years to accept that this is me. But I'm finally here. I accept who I am. That doesn't change anything, except I realize I can only do so much for myself and others and the rest is in God's hands. I will continue to put the work in and accept my life as it is and at the same time try to improve my situation however I can.

Accept who you are and know that you are enough. Take your steps and leave the rest in God's hands.

12. DON'T ENDURE: THRIVE!

Even though I know there will be hard days ahead of me, I don't want to just get through this life. I want to enjoy it! I want to live each day to the fullest. With that being said, I've learned the absolute importance of being kind to myself. If I don't feel well, I'm okay with letting myself rest. I won't beat myself up about it. This may always be the way my life is. I have faith that I will heal and that things will get better, but that may not mean that I will get back to doing all the things I want to do.

Know you and I have great value and worth exactly as we are.

I was reminded of the beautiful necklace that Becky gave me, where pieces of broken pottery were made into gorgeous jewelry. It serves as a physical reminder for me to have hope and that even though I have been broken, I can be rebuilt as something even more beautiful than where I started. Along my journey, I have tried to find beauty and have learned that being broken is not always a bad thing. I must gather up what is left over and polish the little broken pieces that remain, finding the stronger, better version of who I have become.

My hope for you is that if you feel like you find yourself in pieces, I'm here to say that being broken is not wrong. In fact, I think most of us have to be broken before we can truly awaken to the most beautiful version of ourself.

What are you claiming for yourself? What is your beautifully broken battle, the truth you are ready to claim? Come together. Be broken with me. Together we create broken, polished pieces that, woven together, are far more beautiful, impactful and powerful than before our brokenness. We can rise again and thrive.

A NOTE FROM THE AUTHOR

There is a question I get asked frequently from anyone who hears my story when they see me up and feeling good. "So," they start off with, "what is the one thing that has helped you the most?"

Each time I hear that question, big eyes stare back at me while they wait for the magic answer that they hope I'm about to share that will solve chronic illness. I think to myself, *One thing? There is no one thing.*

Each time, I take a moment to put together the best response I can. "Well, the hyperbaric oxygen chamber was amazing and really got me into remission pretty quick. But really, each and every treatment was an important piece of healing for me. It was everything I tried, step by step through medical, natural and emotional healing. I'm not sure there was one thing that helped me significantly because one treatment without the foundation of the others wouldn't have been as successful."

However, as I've thought more about my journey and that common question, there is one thing that has stood out, beyond each individual modality or some treatment that made a bigger difference compared to another. My one thing that has been guiding me along the way is God. During each treatment, each new step I took, I was guided by God. When I was about to give up hope, He would place another angel in my life with something else for me to try, even when I didn't think He was listening to me.

Some people need yoga while others need surgery; it's rare that each person, even with the same disease, has gone down the exact same process to heal. Just as there is no one exact manifestation of disease, there is no "one-size-fits-all" in the healing process. I wish there was a treatment that would heal everyone! Sadly, what works for me might not work for someone else.

But what I do know is that God is there for all of us and if we listen to our intuition and our gut feelings, we will know what's right for us. Nobody else has that power. Sure, people can give suggestions, which can be super helpful, but it is up to us to decide what we need to do for our body.

I have tried many things to help myself and I have been blessed to have a supportive husband who drove me to many treatments. My supportive mom, dad, sister and brother were there for me whenever I needed them, too. My children developed the patience of Job. Recently, I was talking to my oldest girls, telling them how sorry I was that I couldn't show up for them like I had wanted when they were younger, apologizing for everything I wasn't able to do for them. I cried as I spoke to them, wanting them to know that I had planned to be a much different mother to them. Their response back to me was surprising. "Mom," Landan said, "your perspective is very different from ours." Taylor nodded in agreement as Landan continued, "We feel so lucky to have you as a mom; you were always there for us. Even if you couldn't make it to all our activities, we knew you wanted to be there. It made it that more special when you were able to come." I gathered them up in my arms, thankful for the kind girls they had grown up to be. If this is what they had to go through to be who they were, then at that point I knew I wouldn't change a thing. Because each of my kids are amazing people and they became that from what they had experienced. I'm very lucky to have them and other family members who helped me along the way, as well as good friends.

The biggest leap of faith for me was trying plant medicine. It was not an easy decision and I might not have tried it had I not exhausted every other thing before then. Finding the childhood trauma helped me finally connect the pieces and heal, emotionally as well as physically.

Though I've had plenty of lows, I've tried hard to be optimistic through the trying times as much as I could. But as I wrap up my story, I admit I still have bad days. I have accepted the fact that as I heal, I need to be patient with myself. I have come such a long way and I keep getting better and better. Sure, there are hiccups along the way and I still have days where I can't get out of bed. But I have accepted that this is my life and I have found bright windows of happiness that shine through the darkest days and energy to spare on others.

I have found beauty looking back at the hardest moments, acknowledging the strength it took to continue to press on, to keep fighting no matter what. I have found beauty in the broken body that had to be stripped down in order to be built back up again—beauty in the depression I had felt so strongly but am no longer experiencing.

Most importantly, I have God, in whom I have found strength. He has taught me to fly without my feet leaving the ground. I have found beauty in things I never would have, had it not been for all I have been through. I never really appreciated everything my body could do until I wasn't able to do them. Now I appreciate every single thing that my marvelous body can do. When I'm able to walk, go for a hike, hug my loved ones, cradle a baby, serve someone, cook a meal for my family, go to work . . . I appreciate it all.

Brita Bigler Peterson

ABOUT THE AUTHOR

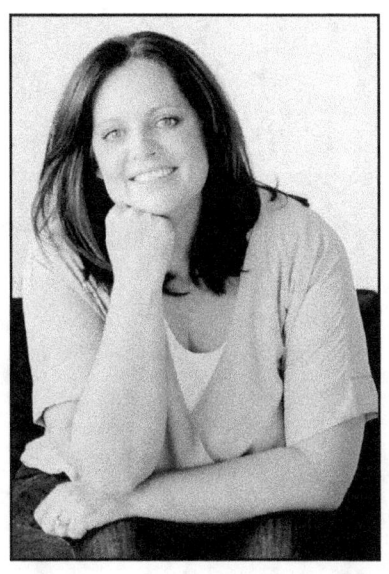

Brita Bigler Peterson is an author, speaker, singer and songwriter who enjoys sharing her inspirational messages with others. She loves helping people that might be struggling since she has gone through physical and mental illness for years.

Her story of healing is powerful and transformational, showing resilience and dedication. She reaches out to those who need her message by inviting them to be a part of her programs and online community, which is a safe space for those who reach out for help.

Brita grew up in a small farming town in Oregon. She has always had a love for creativity and design and graduated from Brigham Young University in Industrial Design. When she is not writing, you will find her sitting at the piano writing and singing her original music. Through her journey, music has become more like therapy, helping her release her feelings as a healthy outlet.

Brita currently lives in Utah where she enjoys spending time with her five incredible children and her loving and supportive husband in their old fixer-upper farmhouse. Family is most important to her and being a mom is one of her most cherished jobs. She loves being outside and enjoying nature and is constantly repainting, rearranging and fixing up their house.

You can connect with Brita on Instagram @brita.peterson. You can also visit her website, www.britapeterson.com, to sign up for emails about new releases, new programs and music coming out. You can also connect with her through email at britabiglerpeterson@gmail.com.

REVIEWS

"A beautifully written book told straight from the heart with honest vulnerability. I admired her faith and determination to keep moving forward. My heart filled with compassion as Brita shared her medical journey. I understood her frustrations as she searched for answers, only to be faced with more questions. I cheered and applauded every time she found strength to push down her fears and face her challenges head-on. I embrace the beauty of being broken, that as we find strength to put ourselves back together, we can become stronger than before. And that ultimately, we might find the courage to forgive even ourselves."
-Tiffani Freckleton RN, NTMC.
Best-selling author of My NICU Story: Written with Love and Letters to a Future Nurse.

"This book is powerful, informative and filled with heartfelt personal experiences. Brita shares her failures of life due to chronic diseases, gained victories through faith in God and support and love of family and friends. We experience her love of sports, hope, and the power of determination. Determination allows Brita to be a winner. However, her life of failing health, and depression created doubt and fears. Brita's faith, prayer, and forgiveness become her source of strength, and she regains her health and happiness of life. Brita's 12 steps for a better life are gems that will guide you a lifetime."
-Toni Stone Bruce
Author/Motivational Speaker
Precious Stones 4 Life, LLC

"I thought this book was going to be about finding the beauty in life after overcoming health challenges. A story meant to inspire those of us in the midst of our disability to keep going, even when life seems bleak and ugly. But what I found in these pages was far more inspiring than a message of "I got

through it, so can you!" Rather, I found a hard-won tale about learning how to recognize the beauty throughout the brutal journey-not just at the end."
- Danny Kutz

"Brita has a talent for sharing the raw parts of her health journey in such an authentic way that it allows her readers to be more accepting of themselves. As you experience her highest of highs, and her very lowest of lows, her ability to take you through her pain and joy in such a vulnerable way gives others permission to move from shame in what they may feel is their brokenness to see the power & beauty that is available through experiencing chronic illness."
-Pualei Lynn
Owner of EDYNKEI Boutique & Founder of ELEVATE Women's Group
https://edynkei.com/

"I was drawn into this book and Brita's story from the first page. If you have dealt with any kind of chronic illness, Lyme or otherwise, you will totally relate to the emotional roller coaster that Brita has been on for most of her life. How she has coped, with courage and fortitude, to get through each day will amaze and inspire you, and mostly give you hope. I was riveted to her story and read through this book in one sitting. I highly recommend it!"
-Becky Peyton
doTERRA wellness advocate

"This book was a great read! I don't have a chronic illness, but I've had some health issues in my life and could really relate and appreciate the things Brita went through in her journey. This book is raw and real! She is an amazing example of pushing through the rough times and embracing the good moments. The message at the end of this book is so inspiring and will touch your heart! I recommend this book to anyone that is in need of a new perspective on hardships, struggles, and life in general!"
- Heather Peterson

"Everyone needs to read this book! Whether you have suffered from a chronic disease or not, Brita does an excellent job of walking you through the full impact it can have on your life in a way that feels so real and personal. I could not put this book down and felt every triumph and pain with her as the story progressed. I feel as if I have now lived through Lyme disease with her to a degree and am so much more empathetic to all that have it. If you have any desire to understand any family member or friend that walks life with a chronic disease such as Lyme, read this book."
-Aubin Palmer
Business and Life Coach
Aubin Palmer Coaching
www.aubinpalmercoaching.com

"What if you lived a lifestyle of beating, ignoring, and reducing your body into a state of chronic illness? In Getting Through Today, Brita Peterson tells her story of living with chronic sickness and moving from surviving to thriving by trusting her intuition and faith."
-Maureen Ryan Blake
Maureen Ryan Blake Media Production

"With a story of persistence and faith, Brita intimately shares her journey, not just of physical healing, but of spiritual and emotional growth. Her words provide a strong and understanding perspective for anyone who's facing their own health obstacles or re-conceptualizing their dreams."
-Shelby Kottemann
2x Internationally Bestselling Author, Intuitive Healer, Artist

www.ingramcontent.com/pod-product-compliance
Lightning Source LLC
Chambersburg PA
CBHW070708130626
46553CB00005B/1898